Teaching Health Care in Virtual Space

To my students, who have taught me most of what I know, especially
LeeAaron Hughes and Courtney Chamberlain,
whose research inspired me

To Anna Holt and Amy Camas, research assistants extraordinaire

To Aaron Beaugh Summers, the next generation
and

To my husband, Fabian Summers, partner and midwife for this project
in every imaginable way

There are other worlds, but they are in this one.

—*Paul Eluard*

This is the first generation of people who work, play, think
and learn differently from their parents. They are the first generation
to not be afraid of technology. It is like the air to them.

—*Don Tapscott*

I never try to teach my students anything,
I only try to create an environment in which they can learn.

—*Albert Einstein*

Contents

Sample Second Life® Learning Activities

Sample Learning Activities Included in the Text

Additional Sample Learning Activities Included in the Appendix

Index: Tools to Use

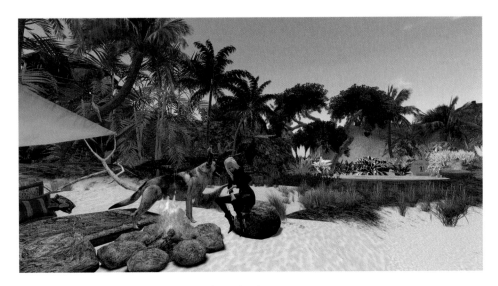

The author waiting for small group discussion to begin

Preface

Why Virtual Worlds?

As long as there has been imagination, there have been virtual worlds. J. R. R. Tolkien's Middle-earth, C. S. Lewis' Narnia, the islands of Odysseus' journey—these are all places well known by readers transported to them through alchemy of word, imagery, and imagination. We know these places by sight and sound and smell. Wholly fictional, they are real to us. Computer-generated worlds are the most recent iteration in a long history of virtual worlds, created by human imagination and inhabited through spoken story, printed book, video film, or computer-generated images.

Imagination is the best friend of learning. When imagination is alive, learning is active, energized, and vital. As new technology has evolved, imagination-fueled learning has become funded in new ways. As soon as there was writing, narrative evoked imagery. When motion picture filming became possible, stories played out through visual images themselves. With the advent of computer-generated three-dimensional worlds, new generations of students can walk, talk, and interact with others in rich sensory virtual learning environments. Computer-generated three-dimensional virtual environments, inhabited simultaneously by many users, are rich with imaginal possibility. There, students can learn business practices by running a business. They can learn genetics on an island dedicated to genetics education. They can practice health care skills by interviewing patients in a virtual hospital. They can interact with patients in a nurse practitioner's clinic or practice interdisciplinary teamwork through interactions with other professionals. These learning activities are easy to create and access, free of charge, in virtual worlds accessible to any student anywhere who has a computer and Internet access.

Why Me?

What I bring to this work is the experience of teaching hundreds of learning activities in Second Life®, a public and free multi-user virtual environment (MUVE) created in 2002 and now used by millions of people worldwide. For over seven years I have had the pleasure of using Second Life® to teach undergraduate and graduate student nurses, other health care providers, non-medical undergraduate students, and interdisciplinary teams. Introducing students and teachers to MUVE learning has become an important part of both my own teaching practice and my research into innovative methods to support student learning.

For Geeks Only?

You may assume that I am a computer geek, an expert on all things computer. Cue the gales of laughter arising from our school's information technology (IT) department! They are on my office phone speed dial. I suspect they draw straws to see who gets to field the next in my endless stream of questions. I am a teacher, not a "techie" or education innovation specialist. If I can teach in the MUVE setting, anyone can do it. Truly I am "one beggar telling another where she found bread," sharing a methodology that has transformed my own teaching and offered my students learning activities that have energized and inspired them. Findings from my own research as well as that of others across many disciplines have provided evidence for the effectiveness of MUVE learning. As I and others "on the ground" who are committed to MUVE learning have discovered, the ease and effectiveness of this novel approach transform both students' experience of learning and instructors' experience of teaching. It epitomizes a kind of learning many teachers have always hoped and believed was possible.

What Is the Purpose of This Book?

The purpose of this book is to present a handbook of best practices for MUVE teaching, illustrated with examples from teaching in Second Life®, the first and one of the largest public (free) MUVEs. Although this book was written for nurse educators, instructors from other disciplines can benefit from the best practices this handbook identifies and describes. The chapters on teaching pedagogy, the history of Second Life®, MUVE learning, orientation to Second Life®, and the problems/pitfalls common for MUVE teaching are not discipline specific. Although the sample learning activities included in the text were designed for nurses, instructors outside of nursing, both those in other health care disciplines and those outside of health care, could easily adapt them for use.

Second Life® is a great teaching tool. It is free, easy to learn, and easy to use. This handbook offers specific, step-by-step suggestions for developing MUVE learning activities and samples to illustrate these steps. Second Life® is referenced frequently throughout the book because it is the MUVE I use for both teaching and research. Most of the best practices described within the text apply to teaching in any MUVE. The sample learning activities described within the text can be used in any MUVE, including Second Life®, other public MUVEs, or private (purchased or independently built) MUVEs. All of the sample learning activities in the text have been used in some form with a wide range of students across disciplines. Readers are invited to use, adapt, and share all materials included in the text.

Sometimes a story is the best teacher. "Talking Story" is a Hawaiian tradition honored at the University of Hawai'i, where I am a tenured professor. Stories of my own successes and failures and also student experiences that have inspired me are included.

Who Is This Book For?

This book is for instructors looking for new and better ways to teach, to expand their pedagogical menu. This book is not for programmers interested in building multi-user virtual environments or creation of land, islands, or structures for use in MUVE learning. The MUVE learning activities I describe do not require building skills or advanced computer expertise. This text is designed as an entry-level, basic, "how-to" handbook for instructors interested in using MUVE technology in their teaching.

Talking Story: How It Began for Me

I discovered Second Life® as I was looking for ways to teach emotional intelligence ability, my academic research focus and primary passion. After only a cursory orientation to Second Life®, I immediately appreciated what MUVEs could mean for student learning. What happened next was unexpected. I began using Second Life® in the classes I was already teaching: physical assessment, medical ethics, advanced pathophysiology, emotional intelligence, development of interdisciplinary teams, and research methodology. My students were undergraduate and graduate nursing students from both health care and non–health care disciplines.

The students' responses stunned me. Students not only excelled in these learning activities but also described their learning experiences as deeper, more engaged, and more lasting compared to traditional learning methods. I gradually increased both the frequency and complexity of MUVE learning activities across all the classes I taught and eventually taught a course entirely in a MUVE. I applied for and received funding to study MUVE learning outcomes. I invited teaching professionals from the University of Hawai'i Center for Teaching Excellence to evaluate MUVE learning in my classes. After one session, the evaluator became quiet. After a few minutes, she simply said, "You are an outstanding teacher in a classroom. However, from what I've observed, your students' MUVE learning is exceptional. I would encourage you to cut back on class time and do more of these learning activities."

I had hoped and expected to see a higher level of learning effectiveness demonstrated by students in MUVE learning activities. Existing research data supported this expectation. What surprised me was the extent to which MUVE learning enabled students to practice new behavior, to make mistakes in a safe place, and to overcome personal shyness and passive learning habits as well as cultural and even language obstacles. With MUVE technology, I could evaluate students' application of course content in simulated situations to a degree and with an objectivity not possible using traditional methods. As an instructor chronically frustrated by the limits of test-taking evaluation, this was a turning point for my own teaching.

Even as I write this, more advanced and commercial MUVE education platforms are becoming available. We are on the brink of holographic virtual environments. Simulation technology will continue to develop, in computer simulation laboratories, online, and in holographic and other virtual applications. It is hoped that the best practices described in this handbook will provide a foundation for use of these future applications as well.

To those wishing to begin a journey of teaching transformation, this book is offered.

Introduction: How to Navigate This Book

Although the historical, theoretical, philosophical, and pedagogical concepts on which MUVE learning is based are reviewed in Chapter 1, this is primarily a "how-to" handbook focused on practical aspects of teaching in MUVEs like Second Life®. The book includes sample learning activities, assessment grids, grading matrices, and step-by-step instructions. Upon completion of the book and review of the appendix materials, an instructor previously unfamiliar with MUVE learning will be able to design, execute, evaluate, and troubleshoot both basic and complex MUVE learning activities.

This book can be read cover to cover or by moving back and forth between selected chapters. At the beginning of each chapter, the "This chapter is for you if" section will help readers with specific interests focus on chapters most relevant for them. The "Reader's Roadmap" that follows describes the topography of the material presented.

Reader's Roadmap: Where Are We?

Part I (Chapters 1–3) focuses on the background for MUVE learning, including the history of virtual environments and the theoretical, social, philosophical, and pedagogical foundations for MUVE learning. This section of the book provides a history of the development of MUVE learning, as well as a description of MUVE learning as a social, philosophical, and technological phenomenon. This history of Second Life® is described.

Part II (Chapters 4–12) presents and discusses samples of general types of MUVE learning activities. For each type of activity, the following are described: purpose, target population, performance outcomes, setup requirements, steps for completing the activity, and procedures for evaluation. Specifics for each type are presented. This is a great reference section for instructors interested in what MUVE learning activities can look like. Sample learning activities of increasing complexity are used to illustrate these descriptions.

Part III (Chapters 13–20) constitutes the specific "How To" section of the handbook. It includes a review of Second Life® orientation requirements for instructors and students as well as specific steps for getting started. Topics include picking the right time to begin MUVE teaching, identifying instructor readiness and a good student group to begin with, and targeting course content most amenable to a successful MUVE learning activity. This section ends with a case study of a MUVE implementation project from beginning to end.

Part IV of the book is the Appendixes, a treasure trove of learning activities, evaluation forms, and other supporting materials that support MUVE learning activities.

Working Glossary for MUVE Terms

Like most exciting journeys, traveling in the MUVE world requires some new language. The chapters ahead will be most useful if the reader takes a few moments to review the following terms, which include both definitions and some additional information that applies to their use. (Note: The terms are listed in the order in which they are encountered in the text.)

Multi-user virtual environment (MUVE): A multi-user virtual environment, or MUVE, is an Internet-based, virtual world that a user accesses via a personal computer. Think of it as a three-dimensional animated landscape in which YOU are one of the animated characters and each of your students is one as well. In this world, avatars can communicate with each other, interact with objects in the environment, and explore by walking, running, sitting, flying, and teleporting from one place to another. This world consists of regions, which are specific locations or places within the overall MUVE world. Some MUVEs are used for online gaming; others are open-ended worlds that can be used for a variety of purposes.

Second Life®: The Second Life® world was the first widely accessible, free public MUVE. Not a game but rather an open-ended world, the user can visit tens of thousands of regions that can be used for many different user-driven purposes. A history and description of Second Life® are included in Chapter 2.

Avatar: An animated, visual representation of oneself in a MUVE. The avatar's appearance (gender, clothes, hair, skin, body shape, and size) can be changed to suit the avatar owner's preference. The avatar's name floats over its head, identifying the avatar to other users. With a few exceptions, every avatar in Second Life® represents a live person who guides the avatar's behavior.

Born: An avatar is born the first day a Second Life® account is made and an avatar created.

Virtual world: Second Life® and other MUVEs are referred to as "worlds." Large MUVEs such as Second Life® are subdivided into smaller areas called regions. In Second Life®, some of these regions are on the mainland of the Second Life® world and others are on individual islands off the coast of the mainland.

Resident: Second Life® can only be visited by a person who has acquired a Second Life® account. Basic Second Life® accounts are free of charge. Once a person has opened a Second Life® account and created an avatar, he or she is considered a resident of Second Life®.

Region: Each region (a locale within a MUVE world) has its own particular characteristics. Locations for learning activities are selected on the basis of these characteristics. For example, if a learning activity is designed for doctors or nurse practitioners, a region that contains a hospital might be appropriate. The builders of MUVE regions often focus on a theme or purpose. Second Life®'s Genome Island was designed by geneticists to help people learn genetics. Regions may represent real places (Paris in the 1800s) or imagined ones (Mars City). As of 2014, more than 77,000 individual public regions were available for use by Second Life® residents.

Inworld: This is MUVE slang that is used to indicate that a user is currently operating his or her avatar in the MUVE world. On my office door I frequently hang a sign that says, "Please do not disturb—I am inworld." MUVE learning activities are described as taking place inworld.

First Life: This term refers to life outside of the MUVE world. For example, "Where do you live in First Life?"

Rezzing: Upon entering a MUVE or when teleporting from one region to another, there is a brief period during which the environment and avatars in it come into focus. This gradual visual change of an appearing object from fuzzy and ill-defined to clear and visually complete is called "rezzing," from the word "resolution." In highly complex and detailed environments, rezzing takes longer than usual.

Lag: A slow computer or Internet connection can cause some MUVE functions to be slow. Environments may rez more slowly than normal. Movements in the environment (speed of a car or plane) may be slow. There may be delays in communication. This is referred to as lag.

Newbie: A newbie is a person who is new to the MUVE world, specifically someone with fewer than thirty hours of inworld experience. Example: If, as a newbie you were to bump into another avatar by mistake, you could say, "Sorry, newbie!" This indicates to others around you that patience and perhaps some help are appropriate.

Griefing: Bad behavior on the part of one MUVE resident that disturbs another resident. Griefing should always be reported and can result in loss of privileges for the disruptive resident.

For more terms, consult the wiki.secondlife.com/wiki/Second_Life_Glossary.

Teaching Health Care in Virtual Space

PART I

Introduction to Multi-user Virtual Environments and the Second Life® World

Have You Ever Wanted Your Students to Experience . . .

- Student discussion groups in which the role and contributions of each student could be easily evaluated by the student, their peers, and the course instructor? Exercises where no student can "fly under the radar" or coast on the work of other students and where air hogs and group disrupters are easily identified and their behavior changed?

- Role-playing that is nonthreatening and low-risk; where feedback is objective, easy, and measurable, so students can identify opportunities for performance improvement?

- The practice of professional skills such as interviewing, communication skills, psychosocial interventions, and peer coaching, in a setting where evaluation against specific performance outcome criteria can be easily documented?

- Group activities that focus on group dynamics such as consensus building, conflict resolution, and group process evaluation, in a setting in which participation can be documented easily and objectively evaluated by students, peers, and instructors?

- Clinical experiences such as rounds, crisis intervention, and clinical teamwork, in a setting in which simulations can be slowed down and clearly documented in a way that facilitates identification of strengths, weaknesses, and skills that need improvement?

- A type of simulation that offers many of the benefits of high-fidelity simulation, without the expense and logistical challenges of face-to-face simulation?

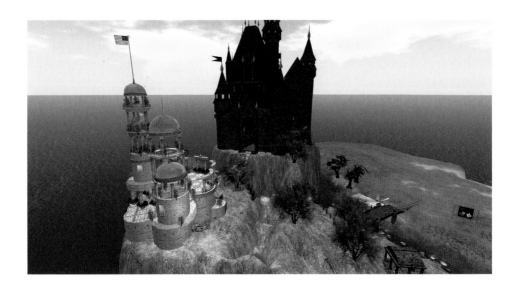

- More efficient learning by replacing "sit and listen" hours with high-quality out-of-class learning experiences?

If so, teaching/learning in multi-user virtual environments may be for you!

Imagine This . . .

You assign a small group discussion for your class. In groups of five or six students, the class will be discussing ethical issues related to abortion. The objectives for the discussion and the grading rubric are sent to the class, along with the location in a virtual world where the discussions will take place.

At an agreed-upon time, each student, from his or her home or other Internet location, logs on to the virtual world website. Each student's avatar enters the virtual world and assembles with the other group members. Tonight, the discussion is personal. The meeting place has been chosen to support an intimate, comfortable environment, a campfire at a beach.

The fire is glowing in the gathering dark of evening. An ocean surf can be heard in the background. The students sit on comfortable seats around the fire. No one looks like they do in First Life, but a name floats over each avatar's head, so everyone is easy to identify. The avatars are not "frozen statues": they gesture during speech, fidget, or adjust their position. Some sit on the ground; others are in chairs or on large pillows. Students greet each other and chat as they wait for the discussion to begin.

The assigned leader for the discussion welcomes everyone and reviews goals for the activity. The discussion begins. Each person types his or her comments and remarks in a chat box. The dialogue in the chat box is visible to all participants. Each entry is identified with the speaker's name and time stamped. Each entry is saved in the chat box, creating a continuous dialogue that will be saved as a transcript of the learning activity.

The conversation is rapid fire and dynamic. There are social exchanges and affirmations. The discussion goes deep fast. It is easy to notice that the group dynamics are a little different. The "air hog" from class is not talking so much. Shy people are speaking up more than usual. It seems easier to share personal opinions.

The discussion ends in thirty minutes. Everyone thinks, "Wow, that went fast!" The group is energized; people linger and talk after the assignment is over. One person copies the discussion group transcript from the chat box and sends it to each group member and the instructor. Later, each member of the group will use the transcript and the assignment grading rubric to complete three short evaluations: a self-evaluation, a peer evaluation, and an evaluation of the group. Participants will identify their strengths and opportunities to improve their participation.

Each person's grade for the assignment is based on data from these evaluations and depends on how each person performed in the group discussion. Evaluations are based on what the student actually said and did, as reflected in the activity transcript. The student's grade is accompanied by feedback and suggestions for improvement that are based on objective criteria and data from the student's performance.

How is this kind of learning possible? How did MUVEs evolve, and how can they be used to design high-quality, accessible, and multidimensional learning that is student focused and evaluated by performance outcomes? To find out, let's begin. . . .

CHAPTER 1

Theoretical, Philosophical, and Pedagogical Foundations for MUVE Learning

This chapter describes the theoretical foundations for MUVE learning. Subjects that will be discussed include:

- Distributed Cognition: A grounding theory for MUVE learning

- The MUVE learner: Whole learning, multiple intelligences, and student power/agency

- The MUVE learning environment: The virtual world

- MUVE learning in relationships: Social and emotional intelligence in learning

- MUVE learning as a societal phenomenon: Situated learning, MUVE as a "Third Place," experiential learning, MUVE as simulation learning, and the role of imagination in learning: the virtual as real

This chapter is for you if:

1. You are interested in the theoretical, philosophical, and pedagogical foundations for MUVE learning.

2. You are interested in a rationale for adding teaching in MUVE teaching to your personal teaching methods repertoire.

Introduction: Virtual Environments and the Evolution of Learning

The argument over use of Internet technology for learning is over. The issue is no longer if Internet technology should be used for learning but rather how best it can be. There is more going on here than the availability of new and more sophisticated equipment. Use of electronic platforms for learning on the worldwide web has caused a tectonic shift in our understanding of learning as a social and cultural process. It also reflects a major change in modern society, the harbinger of a new age. We are no longer in the Information Age but the "Age of Techne"—the creative human online . . . *Homo cyber* (Boellstorff 2008). This book does not defend this evolution but rather accepts it as a given. We are in the midst of a sea change. How, what, when, and where learning happens is changing quickly and profoundly.

Evidence of this is everywhere. Harvard University, a US leader for education innovation, sponsors Project Zero, dedicated to a whole-scale reimagination of learning supported by new pedagogies and new technology. The Khan Academy, founded by American educator and intrepreneur Salman Khan, is dedicated to cost-free education to any person, anywhere, based on Internet learning platforms and new approaches to learning. Within the profession of nursing, Dr. Patricia Benner, a leader in education innovation, has called for a revolution in nursing education. Her vision includes the challenge to contextualize learning using new approaches and new tools (Benner et al. 2010).

The revolution these education innovators leaders espouse has emerged as a product of new understanding about intelligence, teaching, and how students learn. It has also been affected by an evolution in education philosophy, particularly as it concerns instructor and student power relationships. Last, it has been profoundly affected by integration of the World Wide Web and online learning into student processing, understanding, and sharing of information.

MUVE learning operationalizes these changes into learning activities in virtual space. Because MUVE learning is deeply connected with emerging learning theory, it is not surprising that it has been referred to by some as perhaps the most important educational opportunity of the twenty-first century (Richter, Anderson-Inman, and Frisbee 2007).

The Theoretical, Conceptual, and Pedagogical Foundations for MUVE Learning

A comprehensive review of the theoretical and conceptual elements that undergird these changes in education is beyond the scope of this text. It is, however, important to outline some of the important elements that provide a foundation for MUVE learning. To do this, these foundational elements will be summarized using a schematic diagram. In this diagram, learners are located at the center of the learning, imbedded in and deeply connected to their environment, relationships, society, and culture.

The Philosophy of MUVE Learning: Distributed Cognition

Figure 1 depicts Distributed Cognition, a theory about how cognition works. Distributed Cognition is a relatively new psychological theory that posits that

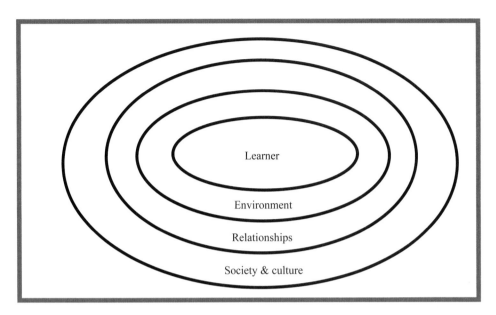

Figure 1. Schema of Socially Distributed Cognition

knowledge does not reside in an individual (the lonely brain of the student). It is, rather, distributed across individuals in a group, interwoven with their environment and processed through complex interactions between individuals, their social/cultural world, and the objects that facilitate these interactions (Hutchins 1995). Viewed through this theoretical lens, social media platforms such as Facebook, Twitter, and MUVES such as Second Life® are integral parts of a cognition system that encompasses the people, relationships, social context, and the interactions they make possible. Learners are intertwined with each other in this network.

This view of cognition as a learning system that includes all participants, interactions, and media provides an excellent foundation for MUVE learning. In a MUVE learning activity, the student, at the center of the learning, is imbedded within a system of cognition that includes other students, the instructor, and both the physical and electronic environments that surround and connect them.

Such a learning system has important differences from traditional learning systems. In a traditional system, the focus is an academic hierarchy located in a physical location. Information flows from the top down. Students, the recipients of learning and at the bottom of the hierarchy, have had little power or agency. The perspective of Distributed Cognition situates the learner at the center of the learning phenomenon, with power, agency, and control over their learning. This is epitomized by MUVE learning.

The MUVE Learner

This new student is a whole being (mental, emotional, spiritual, and social) whose experience of learning is guided by multiple intelligences and fueled by his or her own yearnings, preferences, intuitions, and imagination. Learner agency is at the core of this model. This learner has power and independence in learning. This means that it is the student who ultimately holds accountability and responsibility for learning. Within this view, the instructor is no longer understood simply as a dispenser of knowledge but rather as a midwife and mentor to learning—a creator, protector, and guide for the learning crucible.

This student, epitomized in MUVE learning, has three fundamental characteristics that set him or her apart from traditional students. First, this student is engaged in whole learning. Second, this student comprises multiple intelligences through which he or she processes information and learns. Third, this student has power and agency, in contrast to his or her disempowered role in the traditional learning hierarchy (see Figure 2).

Whole Learning

Whole learning theory posits that students engage in learning with their whole being. No longer considered just a mental process, learning is now understood to be profoundly affected by students' physical, mental, and emotional being.

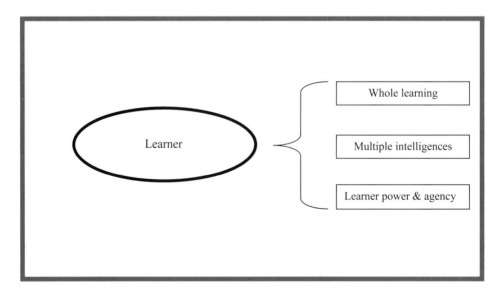

Figure 2. Socially Distributed Cognition: Characteristics of the MUVE Learner

Learning is thus mental, emotional, and physical, truly a mind-body-spirit experience. MUVE learning epitomizes this.

The MUVE learner engages learning not just as a mental activity but also as a physical, emotional, and social activity. Avatar bodies move around the virtual environment, running, flying, touching, as a part of the learning process. The physicality of the virtual environment feeds the learning process. Similarly, in interactions with other students, learning is both a social and an emotional process in which emotion informs thinking as thinking informs emotions. The MUVE learner is a whole learner.

The MUVE Learner: Multiple Intelligences

The MUVE learner also embodies emerging ideas about what intelligence is and how it is engaged in learning. In the past, intelligence was presumed to be a unifocal concept that varied little from person to person. Students were all taught the same way because they were presumed to be cognitively essentially the same. Recent developments in thinking about intelligence are epitomized by Howard Gardner's Theory of Multiple Intelligences, which describes nine primary types of intelligence that present differently in different people (see Figure 3). Each person has a constellation of primary intelligences. One student's intelligence profile is different from that of another student. This has profound consequences for the ways in which students learn (Gardner 1999).

Imagine a classroom with the following students: one who speaks three languages, a gymnast, a Buddhist monk, a cellist, an artist, and a nurse. The primary intelligence that informs each of these is students likely quite different. How they learn may be radically different. The nurse may learn best interacting with others. To best process information and learn, this person may actually require interpersonal interaction. The artist may not need such interaction but may need to draw or work in three dimensions to understand a difficult concept (are you a person who has to diagram something to understand it? You can relate.). The gymnast may tune out of a class in which he or she is required to sit immobile in class for long periods of time. If permitted to move around the classroom while listening, his or her learning may improve significantly. If the cellist comes to class and there is music playing, the music may prime the pump of his or her learning.

Talking Story: Drawing upon the Multiple Intelligences of Students

Two students taught me that teaching with a particular student's primary intelligence in mind can make a big difference. I was in the hospital with a student

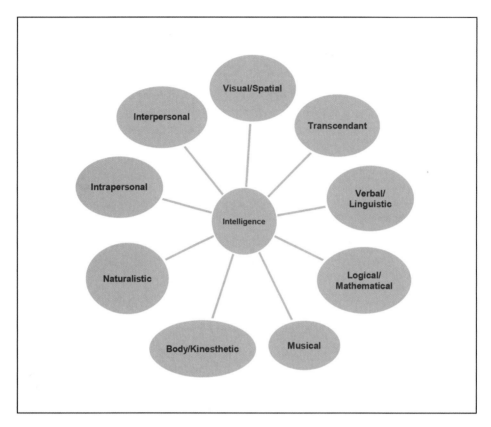

Figure 3. Multiple Intelligences (Gardner 1999)

nurse at the bedside of his patient. The student was performing a procedure for the first time. I was walking the student through the procedure and, as a matter of course, asked a question about the next step. The student froze. It was the deer in the headlights moment that students dread. I happened to know that the student was a basketball coach and inferred from this that he might have strong kinesthetic intelligence. I asked him to close his eyes and dribble a basketball in his imagination. In a second, his eyes flew open and his face lit up with a grin. "I know what to do next!" he exclaimed and went on to accurately answer my question. Drawing on his primary intelligence helped when he got stuck.

Another student stopped me after a class I had taught on multiple intelligences. She was a quiet and reserved nursing student, usually somber in appearance and scholarly in her academic work. When she approached me, however, her eyes were dancing and she was clearly delighted. She said, "I understand how I think now!" She went on to explain that she had always thought in terms of formulas and equations; it was how she approached everything. This disturbed her because she was in an academic program that often emphasized interpersonal skills. This discrepancy in skills troubled her, but knowing that mathematical intelligence was her primary intelligence made her appreciate her own way of understanding the world.

Traditional teaching does not usually enlist the whole range of intelligences that Gardner suggests are represented in students. The intelligences represented by art, music, physical movement, interpersonal interaction, nature, and emotions are usually not considered primary and important means for teaching students. Teaching methods too often focus on a narrow range of intelligences, typically mathematical and linguistic intelligence (reading, writing, and arithmetic). The classical education of the past, which included music, athletics, and art, has in most cases succumbed to financial pressure and at best is considered optional. Students are taught with methods that address a narrow range of intelligences. Highly intelligent students may be handicapped if there is a mismatch between the intelligences the instructor uses to teach (math, linguistic) and their own (spatial, kinesthetic, etc.).

MUVE Learning: Multiple Intelligences Applied

MUVE learning activates a wide variety of the intelligences described by Gardner. In a MUVE learning activity, students are, first of all, in a body! To participate in a MUVE learning activity, a student inhabits an avatar body that walks, talks, flies, and interacts with other students. Learning activities take place in complex, stimulating, and often beautiful natural environments that include both visual and auditory stimulation (a sunset, the sound of water, wind, music). Much of the learning that occurs involves other students, and often emotional engagement is a part of the activity. Such rich environments activate many intelligences at once. When this happens, a wider variety of learners engage in rich and effective learning.

The MUVE Learner: Student Power and Agency

Traditionally, students held a low position on the academic totem pole. Instructors held most of the power and students the least. Within this system, learning was dispensed in the form of course grades "given" and degrees "conferred." Philosophically speaking, education was a paternalistic system in which students had little autonomy beyond their ability to follow rules made by others.

In stark contrast is the concept of student agency. Agency in a sociological context refers to capacity to initiate action in the world. Student agency refers to the capability of students to direct the course of learning. The student is not being acted upon as an object but instead is the primary driver of the learning

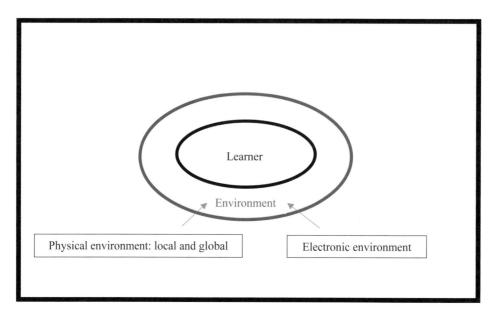

Figure 4. Socially Distributed Cognition: The Effect of Environment on Learning

process. In a MUVE setting, students have agency for learning. They function within the MUVE as autonomous learners, applying what they have learned and manifesting it creatively into demonstrable performance outcomes.

The MUVE Learning Environment

The MUVE environment is rich and realistic, and it helps students envision application of their learning in settings similar to those where learning will be applied in the future. Figure 4 reflects this as the student's local environment is extended into the global environment through the use of an Internet platform. Through its use, students can reach beyond their local environment to connect, interact, and learn with students in a global community.

MUVE Learning in Relationships: Social and Emotional Intelligence in Learning

In the traditional paradigm of learning, humans were considered to be thinking beings who also have emotions. The relationship between thinking and feeling was presumed to be antagonistic. To think clearly, a person had to isolate emotions, which were assumed to have a contaminating influence on logical and analytical processes. Current neuroscience findings contradict this assumption. Analysis of brain function using functional magnetic resonance imaging

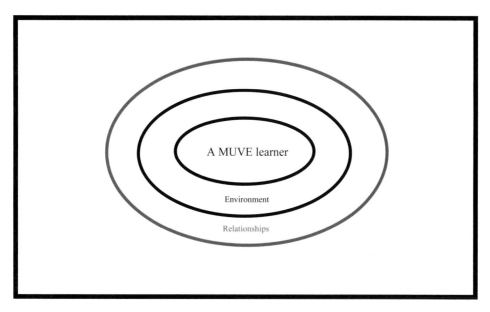

Figure 5. Socially Distributed Cognition: The Effect of Relationships on Learning

and other technologies has revealed that learning integrates many forms of perception, including emotional perception.

The Theory of Multiple Intelligences reflects a complementary, not antagonistic, relationship among types of intelligence. Musical intelligence now is understood to complement mathematical intelligence. Interpersonal intelligence works hand in hand with linguistic intelligence. The emotional currency of interpersonal and intrapersonal intelligences is now understood to provide important value to cognition and learning. Some theorists have gone so far as to suggest that all effective learning has a strong emotional element. MUVE learning uses interactions among students, patients, and professionals that have emotional content (see Figure 5). This interpersonal engagement and the intrapersonal reflective process that accompanies it in MUVE learning effectively draw on social and emotional intelligences that support learning.

MUVE Learning: Society and Culture

Many social media platforms, including MUVEs such as Second Life®, share characteristics of a Third Place, and these characteristics contribute to rich and collaborative learning experiences. The fun, socially leveling, and accessible characteristics of learning activities in MUVE contribute to a socially rich, interpersonally rewarding, energizing experience that positively affects learning. Regulars mentor newbies, and the informal, collaborative, and conversational

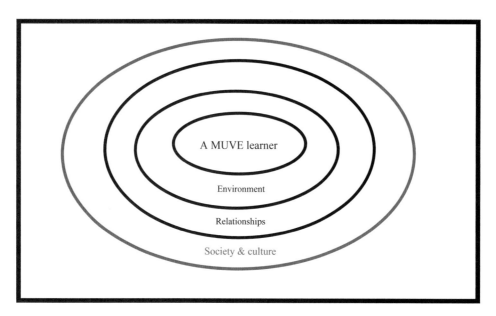

Figure 6. Socially Distributed Cognition: The Effect of Society and Culture on Learning

tone of learning with "the group brain" supports learning that is effective, energizing, and creative (see Figure 6). This may result in improved transferability of MUVE learning into professional practice.

MUVE Learning Dynamics

This chapter has identified the philosophical framework for MUVE learning, reviewed important characteristics of the MUVE learner at the center of the MUVE learning experience, and described the important interconnectedness of the MUVE learner with the environment, other people, and vehicles used for interaction between them. This chapter will now conclude with a brief description of learning dynamics that fuel the MUVE learning system: experiential learning, simulation, and imagination.

Society and Culture: Situated Learning

When learning is situated, it is a function of the activity, context, and culture in which it occurs. In other words, learning is most effective when it occurs as an actual activity in a specific context, connected to the culture and social context that are appropriate for the learning activity. MUVE learning epitomizes situated learning. A MUVE learning activity that focuses on grieving may require students to interact in a virtual hospice environment with a grieving patient. The performance outcomes for the activity can require that the student demonstrate in his or her interactions with the patient an awareness and responsiveness to the patient's culture and social position. The activity itself is in a context that is appropriate to the topic, in this case a hospice facility, in which the student is engaged in interaction with a person who is grieving. In this way, MUVE learning situates learning in the contexts, social dynamics, and cultural environments most appropriate for the learning.

Learning as a Social and Cultural Phenomenon

The MUVE as a Third Place

In the 1990s, urban planning theorist Ray Oldenburg formulated the notion of three primary cultural "places." The First Place is the home; the Second Place is the workplace. The Third Place is the important place where people connect in low-pressure, fun, recreational, homelike places in which community life is anchored in informal, shared experience. These Third Places are considered creative, formative social locations that play a crucial role in community well-being. According to Oldenberg, Third Places share particular characteristics. They are neutral ground and are accommodating and socially level. Third Places have a playful and conversational mood, as well as a home away from home feeling. Such locations are unostentatious physically, usually homey, and easily accessible, and they have regulars who maintain a friendly culture and welcome newcomers (Oldenberg 1999). See Appendix 1.

Experiential Learning in MUVEs

Learning in a MUVE is fundamentally experiential. Experiential learning theory describes student understanding as a recurring cycling of four steps: concrete experience, reflective observation, abstract conceptualization, and active experimentation (Kolb 1984; see Figure 7). Most MUVE learning activities routinely include all four of these steps. A student in a MUVE learning activity could, for example, have a discussion with a virtual patient to assess his or her knowledge about an illness. This is an example of a concrete experience. After the conversation, the student reviews a transcript of the interaction. The student reflects on what went well and what did not (reflective observation). The student could then review course content and theories about communication, using this information to make plans to improve his or her skills (abstract conceptualization). In a follow-up activity, the student can try new behavior to improve upon

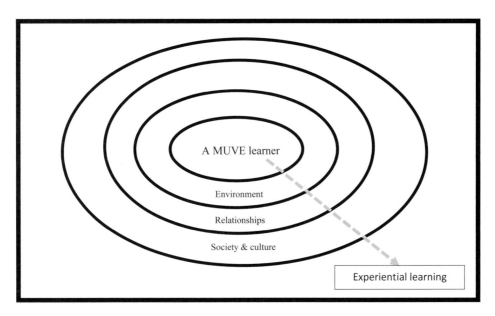

Figure 7. Experiential Learning

his or her previous performance (active experimentation). The cycle continues as the student has new concrete experiences and continues to reflect, use theory, and further improve performance.

Simulation Learning

One teaching method that exemplifies experiential learning is simulation learning. Simulation learning has been used for decades, in professions as widely different as aeronautics and health care. With advances in technology, the sophistication of learning simulation has advanced, and simulation labs of a variety of levels of sophistication are now a part of every health care education program. High-fidelity simulation, defined as simulation that most closely resembles reality, has become increasingly popular in health care in general and nursing education in particular. Some research supports the usefulness of this form of learning, although evidence for the transfer of learning into the clinical environment is not yet well developed (see Figure 8).

Computer-based simulation has been a part of health care education for decades and has gradually increased in sophistication. Learning scenarios, clinical decision-making scenarios using artificial intelligence, and even psychomotor skills such as cardiopulmonary resuscitation and advanced life support skills are used widely. One advantage of Internet-based simulation is its ability to provide learning activities for individuals who either do not have access to

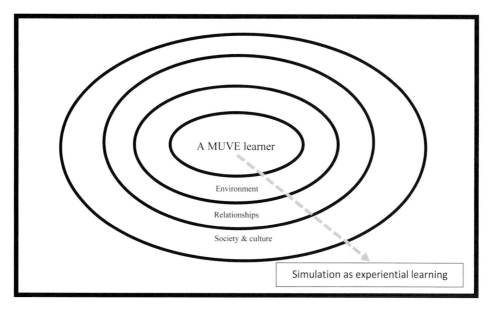

Figure 8. Simulation Learning

high-fidelity simulation labs or are limited in their use of available ones. On-line learning simulation can also greatly enhance online learning and add an element of application and contextualization to this medium.

MUVE learning is a form of computer-based learning simulation. MUVE learning offers many of the same positive benefits of high-fidelity simulation but also offers some things it cannot. Distance learners who do not have access to a simulation laboratory can benefit from MUVE simulation learning activities. Online courses can similarly incorporate benefits of simulation (SIM) without the geographic necessity and cost of SIM activities. Last, even the best of SIM laboratories can offer students only periodic SIM learning activities, whereas MUVE learning activities can be used weekly.

Computer technology and Internet tools specifically do not simply provide improved technical tools for doing the same things we have been doing all along. Changes in communication technology have far-reaching consequences rooted in their impact on people's imaginal capacity. Consider the evolution of writing—from pictograms scratched on a cave wall to cuneiform characters on clay tablets, to calligraphy on parchment, then later to the earliest printing presses, and then from typewriters to word processors (whiteout to spell check!). What an evolution in the technical means for conveying ideas. Far more is happening, however, than the simple transmission of ideas from one person to another. For example, sociologist Benedict Anderson describes that when newspapers became widely available, something profound happened

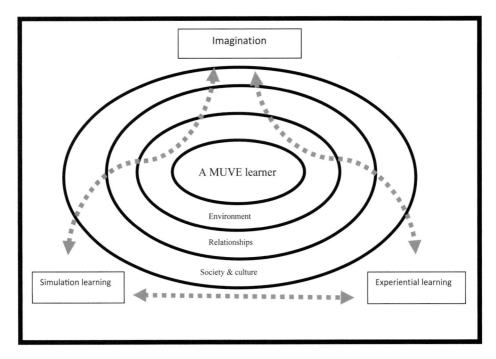

Figure 9. The Virtual as Real: Imagination in Learning

socially. People could read about the lives of people not only in other parts of their own country but also across the globe. This newly imagined residency in a shared global community that transcended geography, time, and national boundaries shifted perspective in many ways. Citizenship was no longer just national but global. People's humanity was expanded, in what Anderson called "deep horizontal comradeship" with others vastly outside their own local experience (Anderson 1983). Through the new media of paper, print, and electronic words, something that was not real became real in the lives of those who used them. This way in which a development in technology facilitated a change in the imagination and imaginal capacity of people was a harbinger of the same type of change observed with the advent of the World Wide Web.

Multi-user virtual environments are worlds where many people from across the globe share residency in a place that similarly transcends geography, time, and national boundaries. This offers the potential for a similarly profound influence on people and learning. In a MUVE, face-to-face interactions happen through the shared habitation of the virtual world. The people behind the avatars both influence and are influenced by each other in ways that shape understanding, experience, and meaning in new ways. There is the potential for imagination and imaginal capacity to lend their power to learning activities through these exchanges (see Figure 9).

In this way, the meaning of the word "virtual" has shifted from its traditional definition (something that is not quite real) to one that reflects simply activity that occurs online. Using this definition, virtual activity is, in fact, as real as anything else that humans do. The technology involved does not determine the reality of what it is used for. Using a virtual medium does not make learning real or unreal. It is the intention of the human using the technology that renders it real or not. In this way, virtual learning is simply learning that occurs online.

Reader's Roadmap: Where Are We?

This concludes the description of the theoretical and conceptual foundation for MUVE learning. Chapter 2 will describe the history and evolution of MUVE learning.

CHAPTER REFERENCES

Anderson, B. 1983. *Imagined Communities: Reflections on the Origins and Spread of Nationalism.* London: Verso.

Benner, P., M. Sutphen, V. Leonard, and L. Shulman. 2010. *Educating Nurses: A Call for Radical Transformation.* San Francisco: Jossey-Bass.

Boellstorff, T. 2008. *Coming of Age in Second Life.* Princeton, NJ: Princeton University Press.

Gardner, H. 1999. *Intelligence Reframed: Multiple Intelligence Reframed.* New York: Basic Books.

Hutchins, E. 1995. *Cognition in the Wild.* Boston: MIT Press.

Kolb, D. 1984. *Experiential Learning as the Science of Learning and Development.* Englewood Cliffs, NJ: Prentice Hall.

Oldenberg, R. 1999. *The Great Good Place: Cafes, Coffee Shops, Community Centers, Beauty Parlors, General Stores, Bars, Hangouts and How They Get You through the Day.* New York: Paragon House.

Richter, J., L. Anderson-Inman, and M. Frisbee. 2007. *Critical Engagement of Teachers in Second Life: Progress in the Salamander Project.* http://www.simteach.com /slccedu07proceedings.pdf#page=27.

CHAPTER 2

What Is a MUVE? What Is MUVE Learning?

This chapter presents a definition and description of MUVEs, including a history of the evolution of MUVEs and MUVE learning.

This chapter is for you if:

1. You are not familiar with MUVEs and/or are new to MUVE teaching.

2. You have worked with MUVEs previously but are interested in learning more about the history and development of MUVEs.

What Is a Multi-user Virtual Environment?

Imagine an animated, three-dimensional world. There are cities, forests, all manner of places to visit. You visit this world using an avatar—a visual representation of yourself in the three-dimensional world. You control the movement of your avatar as it moves through the virtual world, interacting with objects and other avatars in the virtual world. An avatar is an extension of the person who controls it. Welcome to multi-user virtual environments (MUVEs), where whole worlds unfold for discovery and new experiences with new opportunities for learning.

A MUVE is defined as any computer-generated physical space that can be experienced by many people at once (Castronova 2005). MUVEs are three-dimensional worlds that provide sights (a visual interface), sounds (birds singing, crowd noises, the paging system in a hospital), and the opportunity for interactions with other users who are in the same MUVE. Multiple users in these Internet-based virtual places interact with each other and the environment in real time. The three-dimensionality and multisensory (sight, sound, movement) nature of these places offer users a sense of immersion, of really being there.

MUVEs: A Brief History

To understand MUVE learning, a brief history of its technological and social roots may be helpful. The earliest computer video games involved one person.

Improvements in gaming technology expanded gaming capability to involve multiple players. A major breakthrough came with multiplayer role-playing online games. Players competed against each other, sometimes as individuals, sometimes in teams, within a virtual environment created uniquely for the game. Massively Multiplayer Online Games (MMOGs) such as *World of Warcraft* became overnight successes. Players often spent many hours a day playing them. The addictive quality of online gaming became a widely discussed social issue. By 2009, an estimated 1.8 billion people worldwide were using virtual games and other virtual environments online (Digitalspace.com).

Second Life® Is Not a Game

Second Life®, other MUVEs, and MMOGs all involve the occupation of a shared three-dimensional virtual space by multiple users who, in their avatar forms, interact in real time. The environment offers users a powerful illusion of being present in the inworld space. What Second Life® offers that MMOGs do not offer is an open-ended system, the absence of a predetermined narrative. Second Life® is not a game driven by rules or goals. There is no winning or losing. In Second Life®, users exercise total autonomy in their selection of activities and experiences (Hunsinger and Krotski 2012). The only rules in Second Life® are those that regulate inappropriate behavior that infringes on other Second Life® residents.

It is certainly possible to play a game in a MUVE, just as you could go to a park to play a game. But in general, a Second Life® MUVE is an environment,

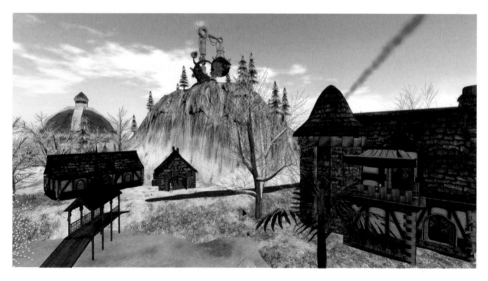

The Second Life® world (huts)

a sandbox, a world where many people, in their avatar form, can meet, communicate, and do things alone or together. There is no specific objective, no winning or losing, and, for general purposes, no specific agenda. One author observed that Second Life® is no more a game than a box of crayons is (Boellstorff 2008). Its purpose is fundamentally different from that of a game. In an apt analogy, Bartle said, "The Pasadena Rose Bowl is a stadium, not a game" (Bartle 2004, 475). Similarly, Second Life® simply provides an environment. Users choose what they want to do in that environment. In Second Life®, a user can meet with a professional colleague in a Paris café to discuss a work project. After that, they could go to a concert in Second Life®, go dancing at a disco, or go skydiving. They could build a house, watch a sunset, attend a lecture, or go shopping. The focus in Second Life® is creativity, communication, and discovery through freely selected activities, often with others, which are experiential, social, and collaborative.

Talking Story

I was teaching a graduate-level pathophysiology class that included a weekly Second Life® discussion group. One of my students, a hardworking nurse manager, was also a busy mom and wife. One day she wrote me an e-mail, saying, "This is how badly I need a break. After my group completed our work in Second Life® this week, I decided that before I logged off, I would go on a mini-vacation . . . to Paris! I found a Paris café region in Second Life® and then spent half an hour, strolling down the beautiful streets, exploring a museum, a beautiful chapel, and sitting in a café for a while, just watching people go by. It was really odd, but I felt like I got that mini vacation I needed." This student had an experience fueled by her imagination, a virtual vacation that provided energy, diversion, and a much-needed mental and emotional rest.

Second Life®

Some MUVEs, such as Second Life®, are free of charge and available for use by anyone with a computer and an Internet connection. Other MUVEs are private and with restricted access. Still other MUVEs are commercial and may be accessed for a fee. Second Life® was the first widely used, public, open-access, free MUVE. As of 2016, it continues to be one of the largest public MUVE platforms in existence. Second Life® was founded by Philip Rosedale in 1999 and launched for public use in 2003 by his San Francisco company, Linden Labs. Rosedale's vision was to create a virtual world in which people could immerse themselves. This was a departure from virtual worlds inhabited by online games.

Early MUVEs were created to be places where participants, in their avatar form, could engage in a wide range of creative activities and experiences. Second Life®, for example, was conceived as a place where people could focus on creative endeavors. After its launch in 2003, it became an immediate success. By 2014, Second Life® had 38 million registered accounts, approximately a million regular users worldwide, and an average of 38,000 to 62,000 users logged in at any given time. In January 2008 alone, it was estimated that users spent over twenty-eight million hours in Second Life® (Wikipedia 2014). At that time, other public MUVEs such as OpenSim had grown rapidly as well.

MUVE Regions: The Landmass of Second Life®

It is the creative role of users that sets Second Life® apart, even among other MUVEs. The Second Life® designers created only a basic landmass in Second Life® along with tools for building on the land. Second Life® residents took these tools and got creative. The original Second Life® world consisted of a large blue sea, a sky overhead, and many islands off a mainland landmass. On these landmasses, Second Life® users created specific regions suited to their design preferences and purposes. Most of the islands and landmasses were (and continue to be) open to the public. Of the over 77,000 distinct regions in Second Life®, approximately 18,000 had limited access as of 2014. Second Life® residents move from one region to another by walking, running, dancing, flying, or, for transportation across long distances, teleporting. It is also possible for Second Life® residents to ride trains, cars, horses, boats, or airplanes (Wikipedia 2014).

Through the creative efforts of many, there are regions that look like First Life locations, e.g., Harvard University's Second Life® Campus, or Second Life®'s Cologne Cathedral. Other regions look like First Life locations in some respects (houses, rivers, trees) but are fictional, created by the imagination of the builder. Still other regions are fantastical places that bear little or no resemblance to real locations. Would you enjoy a zero-gravity experience on Mars? Second Life® residents are free to explore and engage in many different ways the regions they visit.

**Communication in Second Life®: Interactions
with People and Things**

Residents can interact with each other, using a chat box or instant message function within the Second Life® viewer. The chat box is visualized in the Second Life® viewer and can be seen by anyone within thirty inworld feet of those participating in the dialogue. Later in Second Life®'s development, talking via microphone headsets became possible. The Second Life® software includes a text translation function so people who speak different languages

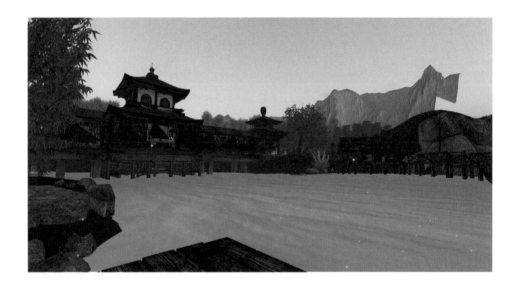

can understand each other's chat entries. Nonverbal communication is supplied with a drop-down menu of sounds (laughing, sighing, crying) and gestures (shrugging, laughing, etc.). Users often use words in the chat box (hahahah . . .) or emoticons to enrich communication with emotional cues.

Avatars can manipulate and interact with objects within the virtual environment. They can pick up objects (a glass of wine, a coffee cup) or wear things (clothes, a pair of skis). They can cause things to move or change (open doors or call an elevator) and use objects for a variety of reasons (drive a car, skydive, or ride a boat or airplane). Participants can go shopping, attend a conference or a concert, or go dancing. By clicking on a movement activation icon, an avatar can move in preprogrammed ways. An avatar on a dance floor could select a dance to "do," for example, tango or wild interpretive dance. In a meditation garden, one might click on a Tai Chi or Kung Fu icon to "do" martial arts. Second Life® users can modify all aspects of their avatar, not only changing gender, clothes, hair, and accessories but also taking on nonhuman or animal avatar forms. A Second Life® account also permits users to make up to five avatars for use in Second Life®. Additional avatars are added by creating additional Second Life® accounts with the same e-mail address but a different avatar name. It is also possible for one user to manage several avatars inworld simultaneously.

The Second Life® Economy

The Second Life® economy is based on currency called Linden™ dollars. Although many items can be acquired for free, other purchasable items such as clothing, house furnishings, and land are available in Second Life® shopping

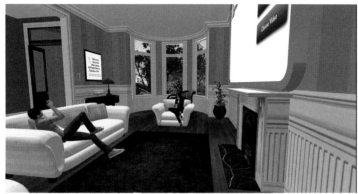

[09:01] Mary: ok, lets get started.

[09:02] Mary: Our task for this assignment is to talk about intelligence

[09:02] Mary: What do you think it is?

[09:02] Greg: That is a really hard question!

[09:02] Mary: Yes—harder than it sounds!

[09:02] Greg: lol

Using the Chat Box for Second Life® discussion

areas and can be purchased using Linden™ dollars. Purchased items are stored in a personal inventory to be used when needed. Employment possibilities in Second Life® enable a resident to garner income by selling goods and services to other residents. Although a basic membership in Second Life® is free of charge, paid memberships come with a variety of benefits that include a home and a monthly income of Linden™ dollars.

Popularization of Second Life®

Second Life® became not only an overnight success but also a social phenomenon. It appeared on the cover of *Time* magazine and was referenced in television shows and in popular movies, songs, videos, and literature. The uses of Second Life® are as diverse as Second Life® users. One of the early social media platforms, it was also used for a huge variety of creative ventures. Art and music are available in Second Life® art galleries and live music venues. Scientists use Second Life® regions for exhibits, education, collaboration, and visualizing research data. Examples include Genome Island, SciLands, and the American Chemical Society's ACS Island.

There are a wide range of First Life business applications in Second Life®. Some of the earliest educational activities in Second Life® involved business administration students who created business plans for corporations they ran in Second Life®. For example, a business student could acquire a Second Life® commercial property, decorate it, fill it with priced inventory, and open it to the public. When visitors select an item they would like to purchase, they click on a "purchase" drop-down menu. Linden™ dollars are then automatically transferred from the buyer's bank account (opened automatically when a Second Life® account is opened) to that of the store owner.

First Life businesses use Second Life® for meetings, training events, and product prototyping. Religious and other interest groups meet in Second Life® in settings as diverse as an Anglican cathedral and a simulated Hajj. Humanists, atheists, and agnostics have met every Sunday since 2006 in a discussion group called SL Humanism. Over the years, embassies have been opened in Second Life®. Countries such as the Philippines, Sweden, and Colombia maintain a Second Life® presence (Wikipedia 2014).

Education in Second Life®

Over one hundred regions of Second Life® were created specifically for educational purposes, including First Life universities, which constructed complete Second Life® campuses. Over three hundred universities worldwide use Second Life® for teaching in some form. Over 80 percent of universities in the United Kingdom use Second Life® in some way. Several educational institutions were created to teach exclusively in Second Life®. Language education is the most common focus of Second Life® learning, but other applications range from health care to business and art education.

MUVE learning in health care has included MUVE learning for disaster response training, clinical simulations, first responder education, and mass-casualty disaster triage. The public health community has used Second Life® for community health education and for avian flu intervention training, cancer and chronic disease survivor education, and simulation of physiological processes (Anderson 2008; Stephens 2009). Chamberlain University uses MUVE training for Ebola education, for learning skills in a high-risk patient population in a safe environment.

Benefits of MUVE Learning

Learning in a Second Life® MUVE facilitates contextualizing learning, group learning, leadership development, precision learning and evaluation, behavior modification, and experimenting in a safe environment. The chat function provides a written transcript of Second Life® educational events (the chat dialogue is simply copied and pasted into a Word file after the event is completed). Second Life® levels the playing field between introverts and extroverts, providing the grounds for objective feedback for group activities that can address the behavior of both air hogs and students who underparticipate. Because course content can be applied in a simulated context that is appropriate for the learner (a nurse applying pathophysiology content in a virtual hospital, for example), learning activities in Second Life® can provide dense learning activities that include application of course content but also professional role development, team function, and continuous quality assessment.

Now that MUVEs have been described and their history reviewed, Chapter 3 will describe what learning in a MUVE such as Second Life® offers both teachers and students.

CHAPTER REFERENCES

Anderson, P. 2008. Second Life—A Teacher's Toolkit. University of Michigan Health Sciences Library, http://www.lib.umich.edu/taubman-health-sciences -library/presentations-podcasts-second-life-teachers-toolkit.

Bartle, R. 2004. *Designing Virtual Worlds.* Indianapolis, IN: New Riders.

Boellstorff, T. 2008. *Coming of Age in Second Life.* Princeton, NJ: Princeton University Press.

Castronova, E. 2005. *Synthetic Worlds: The Business and Culture of Online Games.* Chicago: University of Chicago Press.

Hunsinger, J., and A. Krotoski. 2012. *Learning and Research in Virtual Worlds.* New York: Routledge.

Stephens, M. R. 2009. Virtual Worlds as a Platform for the Virtual First Responder. http://www.slideshare.net.marqueA2/final-sl-for-ed-vfr-03june2009.

Wikipedia. 2014. Second Life. http://wikipedia.org/wiki/second_life.

CHAPTER 3

The Virtual World Is Your Classroom

Teaching in Second Life®

This chapter reviews general characteristics of MUVE learning activities for students learning alone or in pairs, small groups, or large groups. The chapter also includes a discussion of psychosocial issues related to MUVE learning.

This chapter is for you if:

1. You have never experienced a MUVE learning activity.

2. You have experienced MUVE learning but would like to broaden your vision for what MUVE learning can offer.

3. You are interested in exploring the qualities and characteristics of MUVE learning that optimize student learning.

General Characteristics of MUVE Learning

Among MUVE learning activities, learning goals, numbers of participants, and the specific types of learning that take place in them vary widely. Despite this, MUVE learning activities of all types share some general common characteristics.

When I observed my first MUVE learning activity, the first impression was one of autonomous, active, dynamic, and student-centered learning. A MUVE learning activity focuses on students and student groups, who have great autonomy within the learning activity. The instructor's role is very different from the traditional, hierarchical sage-on-stage model. Instead, the instructor focuses on learning activity design and creation of an effective learning crucible. Once the learning activity has been completed, the instructor is very active in the evaluation stage of the activity.

Example: The Evolving Instructor Role

When I first started teaching in Second Life®, I was always present inworld for the learning activities I had designed. I served as discussion group leader and led small student groups in hospital clinical rounds. I was accustomed to being the focus of the learning activity, with the student following along in an important but secondary role. Honestly, I took this for granted. As I continued to teach in Second Life®, this changed dramatically and not necessarily according to my plan. One day I was unexpectedly unable to be present at an undergraduate ethics discussion group scheduled to take place in Second Life®. I asked a senior student, one I knew well and trusted, to take over responsibility for leading the group. The student agreed to do so and the discussion took place. When I reviewed the discussion transcript for the activity, I was shocked. The discussion was significantly better than those at which I had been present. Student participation was more dynamic and the depth of sharing deeper. Student leadership was excellent, and the students had a much more animated conversation among themselves than in the groups I had led. From then on, I offered extra credit points for leading discussion groups. It was a better utilization of instructor time, as I was able to focus more on the evaluation and feedback part of the assignment. The groups performed at a higher level and developed leadership and group skills. It was a win-win improvement in the learning activity.

I experienced a similar situation with a graduate-level pathophysiology class. For this class, one of the assignments was clinical rounds (for a detailed description of this assignment, see Chapter 11). I led small groups in clinical rounds discussing clinical application of pathologies we were studying in class, illustrated by patients we interviewed as a group in the virtual hospital. Weekly rounds were only planned for the first half of the semester. At the end of the last scheduled rounds, I was approached by a student who said, "We have talked about it as a group and we feel that in Rounds we are really applying the course material. We know the scheduled assignments are over, but would you teach us to lead Rounds and continue the weekly assignment ourselves?"

Again, I was shocked. How many times do students ask for more work? I readily agreed and provided instruction and support for students willing to lead the activity as well as for those who volunteered to act in the patient role. In taking ownership of the activity, the students took on new roles beyond what had been expected. They supported each other in learning and performing these roles. An enhanced level of both group learning and group responsibility was evident as Rounds continued weekly for the remainder of the semester. Performance outcomes for Rounds participation continued to improve. By the end of the semester, leadership and case study construction (in the patient role) as well as teamwork outcomes had steadily improved. The group was performing at a far more advanced level than I had anticipated. The group independently took the assignment further, broader, and deeper than I had imagined when designing the activity. Beyond learning activity design and implementation, I spent most of my time reviewing activity transcripts, giving feedback and suggestions for improvement.

In both these instances, my "director and dispenser of knowledge" role shifted. I experienced a new role that focused on creating a learning activity to serve as a crucible for learning. I was able to spend most of my teaching on feedback and coaching. The sage on stage had evolved into coach, mentor, and facilitator of learning.

Active, Engrossed Student-Centered Learning

There is a lot of talk about reimagining health care education. The two learning activities just described are excellent examples of such an imaginal shift. MUVE learning offers an opportunity for students to move beyond a passive learning environment where the student has little power and little agency. MUVE learning places students in a powerful, self-directed center of the learning activity, in a place where learning is active, engaged, autonomous, and focused on performance outcomes. This is reflected in the way students talk about Second Life®. They refer to these learning activities as "going inworld," to a place where they are fully engaged in learning that is energizing and, they often say, fun. One student nurse researcher who investigated the phenomenology of student nurse learning in Second Life® referred to this phenomenon as "engrossment." This refers to a kind of learning experience in which the student is totally focused and undistracted by multitasking or outside distractions, totally immersed in learning (Chamberlain 2014). This is similar to the concept of "flow," in which a learner is immersed undistracted in the present (Shernoff et al. 2003).

Pedagogical Synchrony

One of the most valuable aspects of MUVE learning is the way it facilitates a strategic link between learning activity methods and desired performance outcomes. For example, a learning activity that focuses on communication should involve communication! Students learning about communication would not just listen to a lecture about communication or write a paper about communication but actually demonstrate communication skills. In a MUVE communication learning activity, students perform communication skills and evaluate their performance using the learning activity transcript and the grading rubric. Students can then use these data to articulate specific plans for performance improvement. In subsequent learning activities, they can demonstrate skill improvement based on comparison of self and peer evaluation from the two MUVE learning assignments. Using a MUVE learning activity enables an instructor to synchronize learning objectives and objective evaluation outcomes with their teaching method.

Another simple example is the contrast between a student who reads about cell structure and another student in a MUVE who, in his or her avatar form, enters a huge three-dimensional model of a cell to explore it and learn about cell function. A cell is a structure in a spatial environment, with depth, geometry, movement, and dynamic exchange between its parts. A student walking through a three-dimensional cell in a MUVE learning activity experiences its architecture, moving from one part to another as cell processes do. Using their own physical presence, movement, and senses, the students' spatial and kinesthetic intelligences are activated. In this example, pedagogy and activity are synchronized to optimize learning. (For a description of a learning activity on Genome Island, see Chapter 6.)

Situated Learning

In Chapter 1, the importance of situated learning was discussed. MUVE learning activities are situated within environments similar to those where learning will be applied after graduation. The learning activity context is used both to support learning in the present and also to support translation into future practice.

Imagine nurse practitioner students practicing client interviews in a school lab. Typically, there is a large space and fifty students divided in pairs scattered over a crowded room. In a MUVE learning activity, nurse practitioner students (in their avatar form) walk into a hospital or clinical waiting room, greet their patient (practicing important interpersonal skills of compassion, developing a relationship, and decreasing patient anxiety), welcome them to the interview/exam area (developing the patient's confidence and trust in the therapeutic relationship), and complete the interview (Where do I stand? How do I frame this question? How do I end the interview? What happens next?). By carrying out the learning activity (interview a patient) in a context similar to the one they will experience after graduation (a clinic, hospital, or office exam room), student learning is ideally situated. This not only makes the learning more complex (students have to address issues such as where to stand) but also supports transfer of learning into future practice. The learning is not located in a classroom; it is located in a (virtual) place similar to environments where it will be applied in the future. For these reasons, it is likely that such learning will be more easily transferred into practice after graduation.

Multidimensional, Dense Learning

Another characteristic of learning in Second Life® is the multidimensional quality of MUVE learning experiences. MUVE learning activities constitute dense learning where a wide range of objectives are engaged at the same time. Rounds, the MUVE learning activity mentioned previously in this chapter (and described in detail in Chapter 11), provides an excellent example. During the Rounds activity, students achieve the following performance outcomes:

1. Collect and articulate content knowledge (facts about diseases, lab values).

2. Apply content knowledge (how do these facts apply to the patient they are interviewing?).

3. Demonstrate interpersonal communication skills both with the patient and with each other.

4. Perform teamwork skills that include conflict management, leadership, prioritization, task organization, time management, and building team morale.

In the flow of the learning activity, these objectives are demonstrated simultaneously. This results in dense learning. A lot is going on in only thirty minutes. This is an example of contextualized, multidimensional, and dense learning that not only is highly efficient but also more closely approximates the way that the learned skills will be practiced in postgraduation clinical experience (see Figure 10).

Psychosocial Phenomena in MUVE Learning

A number of important psychosocial phenomena characterize MUVE learning. One of the most important is the phenomenon of disinhibition that students often describe after working in Second Life®. Students report feeling less inhibited during MUVE learning activities. They report less peer pressure, fewer social inhibitions, and a lower sense of perceived risk when offering opinions or trying out new behavior. An example of this occurred in my own experience working with a very shy and withdrawn introvert in a class I was teaching largely in Second Life®.

Talking Story: Teaching beyond the Screaming Extroverts

Education research has demonstrated that more learning activities are geared toward extroverts than introverts (Cain 2013). I had never much thought

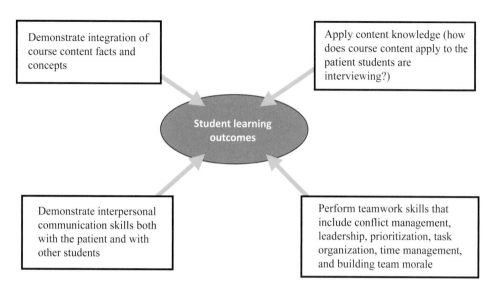

Figure 10. Dimensions of Learning in MUVE Clinical Rounds Learning Activity

about this until teaching a course that focused on developing multidisciplinary teams. This class included students from nine different disciplines, including one art student. This student epitomized the opposite of the interactive, engaged, and socially dexterous nurses I was used to teaching. The art student was a loner, a radical introvert, and obviously painfully shy. She neither interacted in class nor engaged any of her classmates socially before or after class. She answered most of my questions with short, awkward sentences or, when possible, with a nod. She only spoke in class when directly asked a question, and when asked, she looked visibly uncomfortable. Any time I met with her outside of class to discuss this, she sat staring at the floor, mostly in silent tears.

Finally, I suggested we meet in Second Life®. She agreed, and for the first time I was able to engage this student. She answered questions clearly and at length. We began to understand each other. Although she did not change her behavior in class significantly, her engagement in the Second Life® learning activities increased over the semester. Her classmates noticed the change, which could be quantified by counting the frequency and length of her contributions in the learning activity transcripts.

Experiences like this have occurred frequently throughout my years of teaching in MUVE environments. One of the common comments students make in evaluations of courses that used MUVE learning is that shy students participate more actively in Second Life® than they do in face-to-face classes and, furthermore, that the MUVE environment helps overcome personal or cultural factors that work against active participation in learning activities.

Imagination and Real Learning in MUVEs?

The role of the imagination in learning and its power to affect both student learning and translation into future practice cannot be overstated. I first became aware of this in a quite dramatic way after one of my first Second Life® learning activities, designed for teaching medical ethics.

Talking Story: The Bus Wreck

One of the early discussion groups I did in Second Life® (and, according to my current standards, not a very good one) was an ethics simulation that focused on clinical triage decisions made by first responders at the site of a bus crash. Students had to decide whom to treat first, how to prioritize resources, and how to recognize the ethical dilemmas the situation presents. There was a great deal of discussion, difficult choices, and lots of disagreement. As the teacher, I was dissatisfied with the learning activity, but the students liked it and reported getting a lot out of it.

The following week, I got a weepy message on my answering machine from a student who had participated in the activity. "Please call me right away," she said, and I returned her call immediately. Her report of what had happened to her that day gave me one of those spine-tingling moments in which I realized the power of a MUVE learning activity. On her way home after class, she had come upon a pedestrian who had been hit by a car. No medical help had yet arrived on the scene. She described to me her hesitation about stopping. She was only a first-year nursing student, but she reported that she remembered the bus crash MUVE learning activity and the way that the simulation had walked the class through the process of decision making in a difficult situation. That memory gave her the courage to stop. She delivered lifesaving care to the injured person, who as a result of her care survived the accident.

This report was stunning to me. The student did not have any firsthand experience with stopping to render aid. The only experience she had was a virtual world simulation experience. The world in which she had learned was not real, the learning activity was not real, but the learning *was real*. The learning activity, which took place largely in the imagination of the student, transferred seamlessly into a real-life situation, not only on the skill level (how to prioritize and triage problems) but also on the psychological level (moving beyond fear, insecurity, and self-doubt to accept responsibility for care). This story illustrates the power of learning that takes place in a student's imagination to translate into actual performance of skills. One of the important aspects of MUVE learning is its use of this imaginal capacity to both enhance effective learning and facilitate transfer of learning into future practice.

Learning as an Energetic Phenomenon
(Is It OK for Learning to Be Fun?)

It is always interesting to notice the initial reaction of both students and faculty to MUVE learning activities. At first, they think Second Life® must be a game. For students, there is often a sense of guilt (I am having fun! Is this OK?) and faculty judgment (Your students are doing WHAT?). It is ironic that learning that is energizing and fun is immediately suspect! Is this legitimate learning? One of the fascinating aspects of MUVE learning is how often students report that these activities are not only effective and useful but also fun and energizing ("I always feel better after my group does clinical rounds in Second Life®"). After teaching hundreds of learning activities in Second Life®, one of my most indelible observations concerns the role of the learning collective, what I and my students call the "Group Brain." In small group MUVE learning activities in particular, students learn to explore and learn as a group, to support each other's learning, and to use team members to learn, teach, and improve the quality of both individual and group performance. This occurs within the context of a highly energizing, fun activity.

How Can MUVE Learning Improve Evaluation? Evaluating
Student Performance vs. Student Knowledge

Performance Outcomes in MUVE Learning

A serious issue in nursing education is the difference between learning about a thing and learning the thing itself. It is not enough to talk about the importance of communicating with patients about dying and end-of-life wishes. Students need the opportunity to perform this crucial interpersonal skill. It is problematic that instructors do not have the means to evaluate students on the rare occasion that students are able to have such a conversation in the clinical setting. On the rare occasion that a student's clinical assignment includes the opportunity to have this kind of conversation with the patient, the instructor is rarely present. Because transcripts from each MUVE learning activity can be used to quantify performance, evaluation of skills such as talking with patients about end-of-life issues is possible, with self-evaluation and suggestions for improvement included. If students have an opportunity to practice skills like these in a safe place, a virtual world, and get specific feedback on their performance, they feel more secure with their skills with actual patients in the future. In this case, performance outcomes replace "learning objectives" to produce performance-focused learning.

Peer Evaluation in MUVE Learning Activities

One of the most important aspects of one-on-one and group MUVE learning activities is the opportunity for peer evaluation. After a learning activity in which two students take turns practicing a skill such as interviewing or taking a history or systems review, the partners have a unique opportunity to do both self and peer evaluation. Each student can print out the chat box transcript and use the grading/evaluation rubric for the assignment to evaluate both his or her own performance and that of the partner as well. Students can offer objective and highly specific feedback that includes both positive feedback and suggestions for performance improvement in the future. If the learning activity is repeated, students can take their performance improvement goals back into a simulated situation and, again using the activity transcript, assess their performance and compare it with the previous performance evaluation, thus substantiating the improvement in their performance.

The Evaluation Triad: Self-Evaluation, Peer Evaluation, and Instructor Evaluation

Using the MUVE learning activity transcript, students have an opportunity to review the transcript and evaluate themselves against specific criteria (Oh, no! I forgot to ask about allergies.). Similarly, in one-on-one or small group activities, students have an opportunity to evaluate each other and include positive feedback and suggestions for improvement. Students submit the self and peer evaluations to the instructor, who can add his or her own third evaluation and suggestions. When a student receives objective feedback from these three sources based on the learning activity transcript, the feedback is very powerful. This 360-degree evaluation can be particularly powerful in tracking performance improvement (see Figure 11). Because the feedback from a MUVE transcript is objective and specific, the student can use it to improve performance in a follow-up activity. Performance improvement can be tracked over time in activities that recur frequently throughout the course (discussion groups, rounds, etc.).

Portfolio Evaluation

Many nursing instructors express dissatisfaction with current methods of evaluating student academic performance. The limitations of and dissatisfaction with multiple-choice tests as a way to evaluate learning is a serious issue in nursing. Although teaching methodology has evolved considerably, the way students are evaluated has largely stayed the same. MUVE learning offers a different way. The triad of self, peer, and instructor evaluation is an

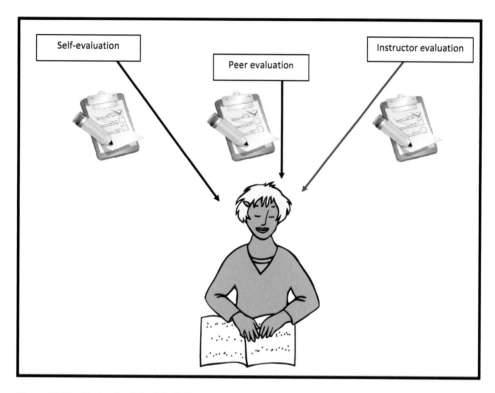

Figure 11. The Evaluation Triad: Self, Peer, and Instructor Feedback

example of a major improvement in evaluation of student performance outcomes. The objectivity and specificity of a MUVE learning activity transcript make the evaluation process easier and more useful than more subjective forms of evaluation. Because the evaluation includes self-evaluation and peer evaluation, the feedback is both easier for students to assimilate and more powerful because it is data driven.

Talking Story: A Final Exam in Second Life®

One of my most exciting experiments in Second Life® occurred when I taught a small group of clinical nurse specialist (CNS) students in a clinical pathophysiology class. Because there were only ten students in the class, I experimented with doing final exams in Second Life®. Each student scheduled an appointment to meet me inworld. The exam began with me telling the student about the patient he or she would be working with during the exam. I presented just a general overview of the patient and his or her presenting disease. Then I asked general questions about the disease and his or her priorities for caring for the patient, based on what the student knew so far. Soon, a nurse (avatar) approached us and said that she was the student nurse caring for the patient that day and that she had some questions about the patient's care. The student nurse asked the CNS student some questions about the patient's care that necessitated an integrated and deep knowledge of the disease pathology. This aspect of the final exam also involved interpersonal teaching and role development aspects of CNS knowledge and skills. The student then thanked the CNS student and left the area. Next, the patient arrived. The middle portion of the exam involved the interaction between the CNS student and the patient. This necessitated therapeutic relationship skills and the demonstration of interpersonal, interviewing, and intervention skills. After this discussion, the patient left the area, and a member of the interdisciplinary team (social worker, physical therapist, or respiratory therapist) approached and a discussion of the care plan ensued (this demonstrates both care-planning mastery and interdisciplinary team skills). Finally, a physician arrived, asking the nurse to review the anticipated plan of care and treatment.

At the end of the hour-long exam, the student and instructor left the area and proceeded to a private but less formal environment to debrief and discuss the experience. I asked the student for his or her perception of the strengths and weaknesses of the exam. I then offered some initial positive feedback and identification of weak areas. The exam ended after an hour, and I subsequently reviewed the transcript against the exam content and skill proficiency criteria for specific grading and feedback.

When I asked the students what they thought of this final exam, several comments recurred frequently: "This was the hardest exam I ever took," and "This was the first exam from which I actually learned something. . . . I wish all exams in nursing were like this." The exam required a lot of trust between the students and the instructor. It was a step outside our comfort zones. As a whole, the students reported that although they felt it was very hard and a bit intimidating, it really gave them an ability to show their stuff. As an instructor, I was amazed at how quickly, clearly, and objectively I could evaluate not only content knowledge but also role mastery and content application. Communication abilities, role, and interdisciplinary skills were also clearly evident. Not only was the exam in context, but I could also see the extent to which the students' knowledge translated into performance.

Reader's Roadmap: Where Are We?

This completes Part I. Now Part II begins, which offers specific examples of the types of learning possible in MUVE.

CHAPTER REFERENCES

Cain, S. 2013. *Quiet: The Power of Introverts in a World That Can't Stop Talking.* New York: Random House.

Chamberlain, C. 2014. *The Undergraduate Nursing Experience with Multi-User Virtual Environments.* Undergraduate Honors Thesis, University of Hawai'i.

Shernoff, D. J., M. Csikszentmihalyi, B. Shneider, and E. S. Shernoff. 2003. Student engagement in High School Classrooms from the Perspective of Flow Theory. *School Psychology Quarterly* 18, no. 2: 158–176.

PART II
Types of MUVE Learning Activities

With Chapter 4 begins Part II of the text, which describes in detail various types of MUVE learning. Chapter 4 presents a brief introduction to three basic MUVE learning activities: solo activities that take place in a content- or context-rich MUVE, learning activities designed for one-on-one interaction, and those activities designed for small or large group learning. In the chapters that follow, each of these types of MUVE learning will be described in detail. The chapters will include specific examples of each type, detailed descriptions for their design, and steps for activity implementation. Each sample includes a description of the activity, target student populations, MUVE setup requirements, activity performance outcomes, specific steps for the activity, and evaluation methods. Instructional notes are included to guide instructors interested in replicating the activity. Specific "How To's" are included for aspects of the activity that require Second Life® skills beyond the basics.

CHAPTER 4

An Introduction to General Types of MUVE Learning Activities

This chapter introduces and describes three general types of MUVE learning: individual learning activities, one-on-one learning activities, and those in small groups.

This chapter is for you if:

1. You have never experienced a MUVE learning activity.

2. You have experienced MUVE learning but are interested in a broader vision for what MUVE learning can offer.

3. You are interested in learning about general types of MUVE learning.

MUVE learning activities can be divided into four types, depending on the number of student participants: (1) solo learning in content- or context-rich environments, (2) one-on-one MUVE learning activities, (3) small group MUVE learning activities, and (4) large group MUVE learning activities. This chapter will describe general characteristics for each of these types of MUVE learning. In the chapters that follow, they will be presented in detail and illustrated by sample learning activities.

Solo Learning in Content- or Context-Rich Environments

There are many examples in Second Life® of content-rich, topically specific MUVE regions. In these environments, students can encounter topical content in lots of ways, engaging and interacting with the region as a means of learning topical content. In the most basic form of this type of MUVE learning activity, a student can simply walk through an exhibit dedicated to a specific topic. In a MUVE garden dedicated to breast cancer education, for example, students can walk through the beautiful space, reading posters, listening to lectures, activating audio material, and seeing content illustrated in other graphic ways. They gaze at a statue, examine parts of a model, or listen to the stories of women who survived breast cancer or did not. This type of learning activity can be a highly effective alternative to reading a text chapter or listening passively to a classroom lecture.

Genome Island is a content-rich Second Life® environment created by geneticists to teach genetics. Students who visit this island are offered many interesting ways to engage with a huge range of genetics topical content. They can walk through a gene forest to learn about individual gene characteristics. To explore inherited physical characteristics, students can mingle with a herd of llamas, changing the color of the mama llama and observing the effect of that change on her progeny. In an exhibit on the history of genetics, a student can walk through Mendel's garden to observe as Mendel did the changed characteristics of pea plants across generations. Visitors to this region can watch generations of rabbits reproduce, watch DNA replicate in a microscope, or interact with a large-scale model of human DNA. In a beautiful outdoor lounge, family genetic charts fly overhead. Students can direct one to hover over their head, available to interact with as a way of exploring genetically inherited diseases. This is a dynamic and active environment for learning.

One-on-One MUVE Learning Activities

MUVE learning environments make it possible for simultaneous interaction between multiple users. This makes it possible to design learning activities that engage students with each other. This type of learning activity is both easy to design and easy for students to engage.

Many different types of one-on-one learning activities are possible. The focus can be anything from content application or demonstration of communication skills to practice and evaluation of new behaviors. The specific environment for the activity can be selected to contextualize the learning. Novice students can practice interviewing skills in a simulated environment similar to that in which they will interview clients in the future. Students of all levels can practice job interviews one-on-one in a prospective supervisor's office or even with a team of interviewers in a clinical or business setting. Students can meet with course instructors in an environment that may be experienced as less intimidating than meeting face to face in the instructor's First Life office. These are but a few examples of the possibilities for one-on-one MUVE learning activities.

Small Group MUVE Learning Activities

Small group MUVE learning activities offer students the opportunity to develop team membership skills. Because group interaction is recorded in the

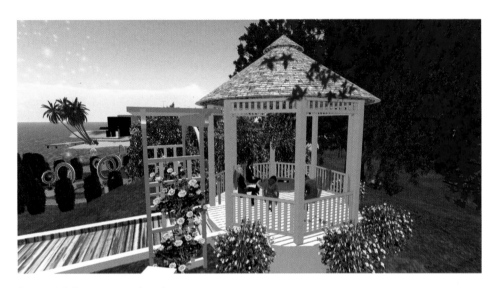

Second Life® small group learning

learning activity transcript, students have an objective tool to evaluate their contributions toward team task achievement and team learning. The simplest small group MUVE learning activity is an inworld discussion group. Others can be more complex, involving multiple students, disciplines, and levels of performance. Team simulation of specialized teams such as institutional review boards or management teams can help students develop specialized team skills. Although professional disciplines such as health care function in interdisciplinary teams, health care education provides little opportunity for students to actually practice interdisciplinary teamwork. In a MUVE simulation, students can practice their own discipline-specific contributions to the team, as well as those that require interaction with professionals from other disciplines. The clinical rounds activity mentioned in Chapter 3 can be designed to include nurses, physicians, social workers, and other interdisciplinary team members. Small group MUVE learning gives students an opportunity to practice, evaluate, and improve their skills over time. The activity transcript provides data that are the basis of self-evaluation and peer and instructor feedback, making the evaluation process objective, data driven, and easy to track over time. Goals for improvement can be made and improvement demonstrated in future small group activity.

Small group MUVE learning can be used at all levels of health care education, from undergraduate clinical practitioners practicing patient interviews to graduate students in MUVE learning activities that focus on professional roles. Doctoral students can discuss and implement policy change, explore research methodologies, or develop new methods of education. Evaluation in these activities can easily include 360-degree evaluations that encompass self-evaluation, peer evaluation, instructor evaluation, and evaluation of group performance.

Large Group MUVE Learning Activities

Second Life® offers rich possibilities for large group activities. An example of this was a conference on teaching in Second Life®, which took place in Second Life®! This virtual conference had all the elements of a typical First Life conference. There were keynote speakers doing podium presentations in large amphitheaters. There were small breakout sessions on a huge range of topics in smaller, more informal settings. There were poster sessions galore! There were also postconference party venues where small groups shared experiences and networks of support and information exchange developed.

Reader's Roadmap: Where Are We?

In this chapter, general types of MUVE learning activities were described. In Chapter 5, the detailed descriptions of these general types begin with a description of content- and context-rich solo learning in Second Life®.

CHAPTER 5

Solo Learning Activities in Content- or Context-Rich MUVEs

The MUVE as a Learning Crucible

This chapter includes a general description of content- and context-rich MUVE learning, with examples of specific health care regions in Second Life®. Strengths and limitations of this type of learning are discussed.

This chapter is for you if:

1. You are interested in exploring characteristics of content- or context-rich MUVEs.

2. You are planning a content- or context-rich MUVE learning activity.

Pedagogical Advantages Offered by Content-/Context-Rich MUVE Regions

One of the most important characteristics of MUVEs is multidimensional sensory richness. Visually and acoustically stimulating, they engender rich imaginal experiences. This chapter will focus on two characteristics of these types of learning environments: content richness and context richness. Learning activity design begins with a strategic use of these two characteristics to support optimum learning. (Note: The Second Life® sites referenced in this chapter were available as of 2015.)

Content-Rich MUVEs

Content-rich MUVE regions provide topical information to region visitors. Such information can be presented in a huge range of ways, from graphic representations such as a huge DNA molecule with which a MUVE user can interact to video and other media. Some content-rich MUVE sites engage participants very actively, others less so. This is well illustrated by two regions in Second Life® that are content rich. Both are dedicated to posttraumatic stress disorder (PTSD) education. At one site, visitors simply walk around reading and listening to information about PTSD. There are posters, family dynamics presentations, and a self-evaluation survey. The site displays excellent information about PTSD in an attractive location that is engaging to explore, but learning there is relatively passive. In another site also dedicated to PTSD, sights and sounds are intended to simulate the experience of having PTSD. In this content-rich site, the role of the learner is more active.

There are many examples of content-rich regions in Second Life®. One such region is dedicated to avian flu prevention. Visitors there can wander through a village whose inhabitants are at high risk of avian flu. The purpose of this site is to provide information about the disease, risk factors associated with it, and prevention strategies for village inhabitants. Another is Second Life®'s Cystic Fibrosis University, dedicated to disseminating information about cystic fibrosis. This region offers information for people with the disease as well as interested health care practitioners. A different type of content-rich environment, POP-CENT, is a Second Life® region that displays information for scientists working on emerging neurotechnology research. Researchers use the site to share information, approaches, topical announcements, and resources.

On a site dedicated to reproductive health, Ovary and Testis Tours takes visitors on a recreation park–like ride in a tour of the structures of the male testis and female ovaries. During the tour, visitors listen to the tour guide's explanations of the anatomical structure and physiological function of the testis and ovaries, which are observed as the ride progresses. Numerous Second Life® regions provide health information of interest to both health care professionals and the general community. Good examples are Health Info Island, which is sponsored by the Mayo Clinic, and its neighbor island, Ability Island, which provides information about several different kinds of disability.

The various MUVE sites described so far illustrate MUVEs that are content rich. The advantages of learning in these regions arise from their ability to effectively communicate content material about a specific topic (such as cystic fibrosis), a specific phenomenon (hallucinations), or processes (neurological research). Others target specific learners (caregivers and family members of people with schizophrenia) who are focused on a specific topic.

Context-Rich MUVEs

A different type of MUVE focuses not on content but on the rich environment within which learning takes place. These sites provide rich crucibles for learning and are valuable not for their content richness but rather for the richness of the context they offer. Context-rich sites are different from those whose purpose focuses on topical content. Context-rich sites do not necessarily convey topical information. The goal of a context-rich MUVE is to provide an environment that particularly supports effective learning. A context-rich MUVE offers instructors an opportunity to match a learning activity with an environment that most effectively supports learning there. These types of sites situate learning within a context that makes the learning richer. For example, a health care profession student who is learning to interview clients can do a learning activity in an environment similar to places where interviewing usually takes place (a clinic or emergency room). Such context-rich sites simulate the environment within which learned behavior will be used in the future. Its richness comes not from the content it offers but rather its similarity to the environment in which learning will be applied. The MUVE is valuable in this case as the crucible for learning it offers and the bridge it creates to future application, fostering translation of learning into practice.

Some of the earliest private MUVEs were context-rich environments. These environments were created as a place to learn a particular subject. Harvard University created a private MUVE that consisted of a nineteenth-century village called River City. This MUVE was designed as "a multi-user virtual environment for learning scientific inquiry and 21st century skills" (River City Project, header). The inhabitants of River City were afflicted with a particular disease. River City visitors investigated the disease by exploring the city environment, the physical surroundings, city records, and historical documents such as photographs and journals. Visitors could interview River City citizens to investigate the source and progress of the illness under study. Working as individuals or teams, students were able to explore both human and environmental issues such as risk factors, infection vectors, and disease spread. River City is an example of a MUVE created to be a learning crucible for a particular set of learning activities focused on a specific goal. River City itself did not teach about the disease or its spread. It provided no information signs, posters, speeches, or presentations by experts on the disease. The River City environment was, rather, a place where students could explore issues related to disease transmission and spread. They could also demonstrate scientific reasoning skills as they investigated the disease plaguing River City. This context richness supported engaged, multilevel, dense learning.

This type of MUVE shares some characteristics with multi-user role-playing games. Students in River City worked toward specific goals and objectives. River City as an environment provided only a context for goal achievement. Context-rich learning MUVEs differ from games because in the River City MUVE, for example, there is more than one solution to problems being explored. The focus is on learning both science concepts and individual inquiry. There is no one correct answer, no game to win (Ketelhut 2007).

Another early context-rich private MUVE is Quest Atlantis. In this MUVE, nine- to twelve-year-old students experience learning through a series of learning quests. These quests took place in Atlantis, a community facing a crisis that arose from poor leadership. Quests included a wide range of activities such as study of the environment, comparison with other cultures, interviewing members of the community, exploration of issues related to social commitment, and formation of plans to deal with the crisis. Similar to the River City MUVE, the primary role of Quest Atlantis was not to provide information about leadership or social responsibility but rather to provide a context within which students could explore these issues. Learning in this MUVE was designed to be very active and included opportunities for both individual and group learning within a context-rich environment that supported learning (Barab et al. 2005).

Critical Life was another early private MUVE created for nursing students. This context-rich site used a specific learning environment, a simulated acute care hospital facility, where nursing students were able to practice crisis intervention skills. When presented with a patient who was in a physiological crisis, students selected the best course of action for treatment of the patient. Their actions triggered specific physiological consequences for the patient. This illustrated the consequences of students' interventional choices. Students could participate either solo or in groups, practicing collaboration skills, learning from each other, and learning performance evaluation (Rogers 2010). This simulation exercise for critical reasoning and problem-solving skills took place in an environment similar to clinical environments in which students expect to practice after graduation. The learning activities involved clinical problems, care goals, and a variety of positive and negative outcome possibilities. When done as a small group, Critical Life learning activities also involved collaboration. This MUVE was primarily a context-rich environment but offered content instruction as well. Patients in Critical Life were programmed to respond to selected interventions in specific ways. When a student performed an intervention, a specific patient symptom was elicited (improved or worsened blood pressure, for example). The students' role was very active, and students received immediate feedback on their chosen interventions. This added content richness to the context richness of the MUVE.

These context-rich MUVEs were created for specific learners and targeted specific objectives. Other MUVEs are context rich but not created for specific topical instruction. Second Life®'s Second Health Hospital, created by the Imperial College of London, depicts a futuristic health care center that provides health for acute and chronic conditions as well as both rehabilitation and preventive health care. Second Health is a state-of-the-art hospital facility that includes an emergency department, endoscopy unit, wellness center, rehabilitation and counseling centers, and a variety of other clinical units. This region in Second Life® is

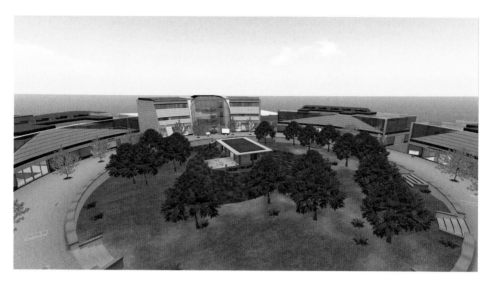

Second Health Hospital in Second Life®

not inhabited. No residents can be found there on a regular basis. There is a welcome sign that introduces visitors to the hospital and a health survey that can be completed. Other than that, there is little content related to health or illness portrayed in the setting.

Second Health Hospital is an excellent example of a context-rich environment. A visitor there hears the paging system overhead just as would be expected in a First World hospital. In each area of the hospital, there is furniture and the basic equipment one would expect to see in a hospital facility (heart monitors, stretchers for patients to sit on, intravenous poles). There are generally no educational displays and no presentations on diseases or disease prevention. Second Health Hospital is simply a place.

This site can be used for a wide range of purposes. Health practitioners use Second Health as a place to practice a range of professional skills. Architects visit the site to get ideas about the design of health care facilities. A patient experiencing anxiety about an upcoming hospital admission can visit Second Health Hospital to practice being in a hospital without anxiety. Public health specialists use Second Health Hospital as a way to explore issues related to infection control. There is no specific content to be learned by visiting Second Health Hospital. It is, however, an excellent location to do clinical nursing learning activities. The clinical rounds activity, referred to previously and described in a later chapter, can easily take place in Second Health Hospital, in an emergency department, a wellness center, or an intensive care unit, depending on the goals of the learning activity.

Sites That Combine Content and Context Richness

Some MUVEs combine elements of both context- and content-specific learning. One acute care hospital region in Second Life® provides patient charts for learning activities that take place there. At this facility, no one can enter any patient area until they first approach a sink and wash their hands. This location provides rich context for learning but also includes some content elements as well.

Another Second Life® region, called the Reality Check Café, similarly combines content and context richness. This MUVE is designed to illustrate the relationship between food choices and exercise. Arriving at the Reality Check Café, visitors are invited to take a seat at the café and to select items from a menu on the table. After indicating their choices, visitors are given a calorie summary of their order. Next, the visitors are invited across the street to a fitness center, where a wide range of exercise machines are available. Once the visitors select one for use and begin to exercise (on a treadmill, exercise bicycle, or other piece of exercise equipment), they are informed about the length of time they will need to exercise to metabolize all the calories generated by their café menu choices. This MUVE uses the context of a café and a fitness center to teach about healthy food and exercise choices. In addition to situating learning in an environment specific to the learning goal (restaurant and fitness center), the specific caloric consequences of food and exercise choices contribute a content focus to this MUVE. This site is a good example of a MUVE that is both context rich and content rich.

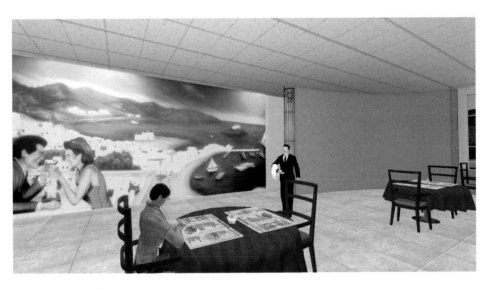

Reality Check Café in Second Life®

The University of Kansas also sponsors a Second Life® MUVE site for medical professionals that combines content and context richness, called the Medical Examiner's Office. This MUVE illustrates a medical examiner's office where visitors can observe autopsies, attend lectures, and interact with equipment and protective clothing typical of such an office. Because this site is also a place for medical professionals to perform learning activities, it also combines content richness with context richness.

Some MUVEs combine context richness and content richness through the use of robot teachers that are programmed to inhabit the MUVE. These robot avatars are not associated with a live user but rather are preprogrammed parts of the MUVE environment. They are designed to interact with site participants, who click on the robot to activate it. An example of this is a Second Life® intensive care unit where visitors interact with preprogrammed robot patients. Visitors observe physiological data provided by the robot patient and make adjustments in medications and other medical treatments. The robot avatar patient is preprogrammed to respond in specific ways to these interventions. Students learn both by observing the patient in situ and by observing patient responses to medical interventions. In other MUVEs, preprogrammed avatar robots are used as avatar coaches who give site visitors feedback about their learning activity performance. What all these examples have in common is the way they combine content and context richness to support learning.

Pedagogical Benefits of Context- and Content-Rich MUVEs

Learning MUVEs that are content or context rich offer several pedagogical benefits. Participants have freedom to explore, to problem solve, and to experience both learning content and process directly. Students engage with information that pertains to their interests. Learning is thus student driven. This experiential focus enables participants to create and develop meaning constructs that help them to expand and deepen their understanding.

For example, participants in River City arrive in the city with no idea of how to look for a disease. They might begin by exploring the physical surroundings, perhaps observing environmental contaminants. Later they might interview River City residents ("Everyone is too afraid to go to the doctor"). Students construct ideas about investigating disease outbreaks and factors specific to new disease transmission. They explore factors that make this search difficult (fear and lack of information). At the Second Life® Virtual Hallucinations region, participants might have experiences that assist them in understanding patients who have auditory or visual hallucinations ("I realized I had no reliable frame of reference. I had no way of knowing what was real and what was not.").

Limitations of Environment as Pedagogy

A significant disadvantage of a content/context-rich type of MUVE learning is that such regions are time, energy, and resource intensive to build. If an instructor decides to create a content- or context-rich MUVE, a high degree of technological expertise or expert assistance is needed. Most instructors do not have these resources and choose to focus on designing and implementing learning activities.

Most topic-specific MUVE learning environments, even the most complex and detailed ones, present highly focused learning of a relatively small body of knowledge. The hallucinations MUVE is very effective, but it only engages a very small segment of a very large topic. For some purposes, this is not a serious limitation. One of the early uses of the University of Hawai'i (UH) Second Life® campus was for automobile drivers' education. The earliest UH Second Life® campus had a track around it, which was used to practice safe driving skills. As psychomotor skills go, driving skills are fairly limited in number and complexity, but for most topics, that is not the case.

Another weakness of teaching in content/context-rich MUVEs is that, like all experiential learning, MUVE learning offers students an opportunity to create their own meaning constructs. This type of learning is sometimes criticized for having vague or poorly defined learning outcomes. Specific goals and performance outcomes may be more difficult to achieve using learning activities that focus on a student's own creation of meaning systems. Designers of learning activities for content- and context-rich MUVEs must understand this challenge and incorporate learning specificity into the instructional design.

Reader's Roadmap: Where Are We?

In this chapter, general characteristics, pedagogical advantages, and disadvantages of content- and context-rich MUVE learning have been discussed. In Chapter 6, two specific examples of these types of learning activities will be presented.

CHAPTER REFERENCES

Barab, S., M. Thomas, T. Dodge, R. Carteaux, and H. Tuzun. 2005. Making Learning Fun: Quest Atlantis, a Game without Guns. *Educational Technology Research and Development* 53, no. 1: 86–107.

Ketelhut, D. J. 2007. The Impact of Student Self-Efficacy on Scientific Inquiry Skills: An Exploratory Investigation of River City, a Multi-user Virtual Environment. *Journal of Science Education and Technology* 16, no. 1: 99–111.

Rogers, L. 2011. Developing Simulations in Multi-User Virtual Environments to Enhance Healthcare Education. *British Journal of Educational Technology* 42, no. 4: 608–615.

CHAPTER 6

Sample Learning Activities 1–3

Solo Learning in Content- or Context-Rich MUVEs

In this chapter, specific learning activities are described that serve as examples of MUVE learning in content- and context-rich learning environments. For each sample, the following will be described: the activity purpose, target population, performance outcomes, MUVE setup requirements, activity procedures, and evaluation options.

This chapter is for you if:

1. You are interested in a specific example of a learning activity in a content- and/or context-rich environment.

2. You are interested in MUVE learning activities specific to genetics.

Introduction to Sample Learning Activities
1 and 2: Genome Island

This book is full of examples of ways to use content- and context-rich MUVEs. One excellent example of a site that provides both is Genome Island, a Second Life® site built by genetics professionals at Texas Wesleyan University to teach genetics. The island is content rich, offering a wide range of ways to learn about genetics. Students can walk through a chromosome forest to learn about characteristics of individual genes. They can go to the genetics lab and look through microscopes to see DNA replicating. Visitors can explore the Gene Pool that illustrates antibiotic resistance.

Talking Story: Discussion Group on Genome Island

As well as being a content-rich environment, Genome Island is also context rich. Students often feel intimidated by the complexity of genetics, so I often use the beauty of the environment as a place for discussion group to offset this. I meet with small groups of students in the open-air Genetics Lab lounge, located on a beautiful open-air porch. We sit in beanbag chairs, and as we sit, family genome charts fly by overhead. Students can say, "Grab that one!" and someone in the group clicks on one of the charts, which then hovers over the group. We can then use it as a focus for discussion. I can click on various parts of the chart to modify it for discussion purposes. A veritable feast of active experiential learning!

The following learning activities offer very simple uses of Genome Island as a content-rich MUVE. They focus on the region's content and context richness.

Sample Learning Activity 1: The Genome Island Postcard

Introduction and Purpose

Genetics can be an intimidating topic for some students, so I often begin the genetics module for my advance pathophysiology course with a learning activity in which students explore Genome Island. The purpose of this learning activity is to facilitate exploration of the Genome Island region and to serve as an introduction to learning genetics in a MUVE setting. This assignment direct students to "go learn something on Genome Island." In Second Life®, a student can click on the "send a postcard" icon, which will take a picture of what the student is doing at that moment. The student can add a message to the picture postcard and send it to a specific e-mail address. Students for the Genome Island assignment report on the outcome of their learning activity by e-mailing the instructor a Second Life® postcard. (See "Tools to Use" below.)

Target Population

This assignment is appropriate for any student population. In this chapter, it is used to illustrate a solo learning assignment, but it can also be used effectively for one-on-one or small group learning activities as well.

Performance Outcomes

Students will demonstrate independent learning by exploring Genome Island and sending the instructor a postcard to describe one learning experience they had there.

MUVE Setup

There are no MUVE setup requirements for this learning activity other than a general orientation to Second Life®.

Activity Procedures

Assignment: Students spend thirty minutes in Second Life®, on Genome Island, exploring the island and the variety of genetics learning that is possible there. After completing Second Life® orientation requirements, students will:

1. Receive a description of the learning activity requirements and instructions on how to take a postcard in Second Life®.

2. Spend thirty minutes in Second Life®, on Genome Island, exploring the island.

3. Identify one area of the region where they learned something interesting.

4. Identify one thing they learned while exploring that region.

5. Take a postcard picture (see below) of themselves and, on the postcard, describe what they learned.

6. Send the postcard to the instructor.

Evaluation

Because of the simplicity and basic introductory nature of this assignment, there are no specific evaluation methods suggested. This can easily be a pass/fail assignment. If portfolio evaluation is used for the course, the student can print out a copy of the e-mail sent to the instructor to include in the portfolio.

Talking Story: Using Second Life® Postcards

During one semester when I used this learning activity to introduce genetics course content, I received a postcard from a student in my class. "I wanted to learn about cells," she said on a postcard picture of her standing next to a huge three-dimensional cell. "But I had to ask myself, 'How do things get into cells, anyway?'" She reported her success in entering the cell and continued with a description of what she had learned about semipermeable membranes and active transport. I was pleased but then surprised to get a second and third postcard from the same student. The assignment required only one postcard! She was so excited about what she learned that she sent postcards of herself sitting on a mitochondria, observing its enzymatic activity, and later another about her frustrating attempts to leave the cell. This active engagement with cellular mechanics clearly energized her and left her wanting more.

Tools to Use: How to Send a Postcard in Second Life®

1. In Second Life®, arrange the scene you would like depicted in the postcard.

2. On the left-hand side of the Second Life® viewer, click on the icon that looks like a camera.

3. A drop-down menu of camera options will appear. Click on the e-mail option.

4. The e-mail setup will appear. The image that will appear in the e-mail is at the top of the setup screen. If satisfied with the picture, enter the e-mail address of the recipient, a title for the message, and any message to be added.

5. Click "send."

6. The postcard will be sent to the recipient's e-mail address.

Sample Learning Activity 2: The Genome Island Treasure Hunt

Introduction and Purpose

The purpose of the Genome Island treasure hunt is to give students an opportunity to identify the genetics resources available on Genome Island by having them complete a treasure hunt checklist using a list of items to be found on Genome Island. At each location, a short assignment invites exploration of one of the following issues: the genetic basis for antibiotic resistance, the genetic foundation for disease, family patterns of disease transmission, and gene dominance.

Target Population

Although most commonly used for individual learning activities, content-rich environments also can be used for pairs or small group learning activities. This learning activity works best as an assignment for students alone or in pairs.

Performance Outcomes

Upon completion of the learning activity, students will be able to:

1. Identify chromosomal abnormalities associated with five common diseases.

2. Describe eight types of genetic disease transmission.

3. Analyze characteristics of progeny anticipated from a series of crosses of dominant and recessive genes.

4. Describe the genetic phenomena of antibiotic resistance and explain why completion of a prescribed antibiotic regimen is important for antibiotic resistance prevention.

MUVE Setup

One advantage of this type of learning activity is the lack of any specific setup or preparation requirements. Students should be sent directions for the activity, including its goals, objectives, and grading rubric, as well as directions for how to get to the Second Life® region where the learning activity will take place. Beyond this, little setup for the activity is required.

Activity Procedures

Note: all activity steps outlined for the remainder of the text assume that the students have completed the Second Life® orientation.

Instructor steps: Orient the students to the activity and create a grading matrix for the assignment; distribute both to students.

Student steps:

1. Go to Genome Island.

2. At the landing area, click on "Teleport to the gene pool."

3. Once you arrive at the gene pool, walk into the pool (you will be under water).

4. In the gene pool, you will find a box labeled "microorganisms."

5. Click on the box and click on "keep the notecard."

6. The notecard that opens gives directions on what to do next.

7. Complete the activity and write a short answer to the following question: What is antibiotic resistance, how does it happen, and what does it have to do with the importance of completing prescribed courses of antibiotics?

8. Return to the laboratory tower and climb to level nine. There you will find models of chromosomes. Click on each one and read the card associated with each. Your goal is to identify five common diseases and the chromosomal abnormality associated with each one.

9. Climb to level ten and identify the type of genetic transmission associated with the eight family genome charts on the poster about genetic transmission.

10. Locate Mendel's garden and proceed to the greenhouse. Play "The Mating Game" and describe the results of dominant and recessive pairings that you create. Describe the results in a paragraph.

Evaluation

Evaluation of the learning activity uses an evaluation rubric specific to the intended performance outcomes. Surveys and quizzes offered in some topical sites can be used for evaluation as well. Postcards and other self-reflective reports of the student's time inworld can be used for evaluation, particularly for reflection activities. For this learning activity, the instructor can select aspects of the activity for grading. A sample for one grading rubric is included in Appendix 9.

Sample Learning Activity 3: Scientific Evaluation of Herbal Preparations

Introduction and Purpose

This learning activity offers students the opportunity to explore a content-rich learning environment in Second Life®. The purpose of this learning activity is to introduce students to scientific evaluation of medicinal use of herbs.

Target Population

This assignment is appropriate for any student population. In this chapter, it is used as a solo learning assignment.

Performance Outcomes

By the end of the thirty-minute learning activity, students will be able to:

1. Describe criteria for the scientific (research-based) evaluation of the use of herbs for medicinal properties.

2. Describe two traditions through which herbal medicines can be evaluated.

3. Describe the evidence-based uses of five herbs, citing both the use of the herb and the evidence that supports its use.

MUVE Setup

This learning activity takes place on Health Information Island, a site sponsored by the Mayo Clinic. Other than directions for how to reach the island, there are no MUVE setup requirements for this learning activity.

Activity Procedures

1. Students are assigned to spend thirty minutes on Second Life's® Health Information Island.

2. After arrival at the landing area, students are asked to proceed to the herb garden, which can be seen a short distance from the landing area.

3. At the herb garden, students are asked to take a notecard from the sign next to the garden that offers information from previous presentations about herbs. (See the end of this chapter: "Tools to Use: How to Accept a Notecard or Other Object.")

4. After this is completed, the student is asked to sit in front of the large screen and read through the presentations. (See the end of this chapter: "Tools You Can Use: How to Watch a Presentation in Second Life®.")

5. After watching the presentation, students will identify the criteria by which evidence supporting use of herbs is evaluated, describing two traditions within which herbal use can be evaluated and citing the scientific evidence for use of five herbs, including indications for their use. This assignment is sent to the instructor in a Word file at the end of the learning activity.

Evaluation

This learning activity is relatively simple to evaluate, as it is a fact-based assignment that can be graded according to a grading rubric created by the instructor.

Tools to Use: How to Accept a Notecard or Other Object

While exploring a content-rich environment, visitors are often offered notecards that contain information that is useful or informative. Many times, a card is offered in a popup screen that the visitor can use to accept or discard the offer. At Health Information Island's Herb Garden, there is a sign next to the garden that invites visitors to receive a notecard that includes information about the medicinal use of herbs.

1. Right click on the sign.

2. Select the drop-down choice to accept the notecard.

3. Once you have accepted the card, look to the far left-hand side of your Second Life® viewer, and click on the suitcase (this is the icon for all the items in storage in your inventory).

4. Your inventory will open, with a range of headings (clothes, objects, notecards). This particular notecard is located under "objects." Scroll down until you find it and click on it, and the notecard screen will open with information about herbs and medicinal use of plants.

Tools to Use: How to Watch a Presentation in Second Life®

A wide variety of presentations are available in Second Life®. Some of these are live presentations given by residents who are sharing information with others in conference venues, academic settings, and other public presentation locations. Other presentations are programmed into a content-rich site as a medium for engaging information. These can take several forms. In the simplest form, such as that represented by the Herbal Medicines presentation, there is a presentation area that consists of a viewing screen and chairs. Watching the presentation is as simple as sitting down in front of the screen and clicking on the screen arrows to advance the slides of the presentation.

Other presentations are more involved, but all have the three elements just illustrated: a viewing screen (which shows anything from PowerPoint slides to video with audio), a sitting area for the avatar, and a means to start and control the presentation.

Reader's Roadmap: Where Are We?

In this chapter, several simple examples of MUVE learning activities in content/context-rich environments have been presented. In Chapter 7, characteristics of MUVE small group learning activities will be described.

CHAPTER 7

Pedagogical Benefits of One-on-One MUVE Learning Activities

This chapter discusses the pedagogical benefits of one-on-one MUVE learning. This chapter is for you if:

1. You are interested in exploring obstacles to learning that a one-on-one MUVE format helps students overcome.

2. You are interested in exploring characteristics of one-on-one MUVE learning activities.

Pedagogical Benefits of One-on-One Learning: Overcoming Social Obstacles to Learning

A variety of interpersonal social dynamics can present serious obstacles to student learning. Such obstacles may arise in any student learning that involves interpersonal interactions but are particularly evident when the learning is one-on-one. This chapter describes some ways in which MUVE learning helps students overcome these obstacles, including social inhibition, language barriers, challenges of high-risk learning situations, and learning that is disruptive.

Overcoming Social Inhibition

A variety of factors can make students feel inhibited in learning activities that involve interactions with other students. This is particularly true in the intimacy of one-on-one interactions. The MUVE learning format can be a powerful tool for helping students overcome such inhibitions. Students familiar with MUVE learning report a phenomenon called disinhibition. Students often report that they felt freer to participate in the MUVE activity than in other forms of learning they have experienced in the past. Shy students often report feeling less self-conscious and less inhibited when they are interacting with others through their avatar form. They report finding it easier to express themselves, to state their own ideas, and to disagree with those of others. One student said, "When I am talking to another person face-to-face, it is hard for me to say what I really think. In the MUVE activity, my classmates listen to me but they are not in my face. That made it easier to say what I really think." Students also report feeling freer to try new behavior, to act outside their comfort zone. They find communicating in the MUVE setting easier because they feel freer from the negative effects of peer pressure, self-consciousness, or negative nonverbal partner behaviors. In MUVE learning activities, participants are one step removed from face-to-face interactions. This space makes interactions and learning easier and more effective.

Disinhibition is important for students in other ways. Students who have difficulty communicating or are socially awkward similarly report feeling less inhibited and more effective in the MUVE environment. When offered the choice between face-to-face activities and the same assignment in a MUVE, many such students prefer the MUVE assignment. Students who experience gender or cultural obstacles similarly report feeling more comfortable speaking through their MUVE avatar. Trying out new behavior in this setting feels safer and easier. "In Second Life®, I came out of my shell," one student reported. "I could be the person I want to be." This student went on to say that her family and friends had noticed and commented on a change in her First Life behavior. The student attributed this to her experience practicing new behaviors—in her words, "Being the way I want to be." In this case, her Second Life® behavior translated into her First Life behavior.

Successfully Managing Relationships Where There Is a High Power Differential

Student learning can be difficult in face-to-face interactions in which there is a power differential. This problem can occur in any relationship where one person perceives that the other person has more power. Although the most obvious example for students occurs in relationships with instructors, such perceived power differentials can occur between students as well. When students feel that they have less power than the person they are interacting with, they may not feel comfortable saying what they really think, stating what they don't understand, or expressing opinions that contradict those others.

Cultural issues can contribute to this dynamic. In some cultures, students who express different opinions from those of their instructor are considered disrespectful. In such cultures, even expressing a lack of understanding can be considered a negative reflection on the instructors' teaching ability. Students may thus feel uncomfortable in a coaching or mentoring relationship with an instructor whom the student perceives as very powerful. Students who are intimidated by people in power or who feel insecure interacting with those in power may also have difficulty accessing the tremendous creativity and power of mentoring or coaching relationships. All these examples of difficulty in power differential relationships can result in obstacles to effective learning. In MUVE learning activities, the disinhibition phenomenon described above can mitigate potentially disruptive effects of face-to-face activities that involve power differential relationships. For professionals for whom power differential relationships are common, this learning can assist students with developing necessary skills.

Talking Story: How Intimidating Can a Cartoon Character Be?

Although my avatar is professionally distinct (dressed in a business suit and tie), I am often amused to notice that when I meet inworld with students for a learning activity, they invariably greet me less formally than they do in class. They are also often both chatty and highly interactive, even students who are shy in person. I also notice that I seem to be able to push students harder and at times be more confrontational without disrupting the learning relationship. I have come to realize that many students find it easier to relate to me in my avatar form. How intimidating can a cartoon character be? In this case, interacting in a MUVE seems to mitigate problems related to the power differential between instructor and students. The MUVE setting works against power differential inhibitions between students and instructor in a way that facilitates learning in general and particularly the mentoring and coaching aspect of the student-teacher relationship.

Overcoming Language Barriers

Learning can be particularly difficult when English is not a student's first language. This can be particularly challenging in one-on-one learning activities. Students for whom English is a second language (ESL) often report that MUVE learning makes it easier for them to participate in learning activities that involve one-on-one and small group formats. Because the dialogue in MUVE learning activities is typed into a chat box, these students have the opportunity to visualize the dialogue. Instead of listening and translating, they are reading and translating. They report that this makes it easier for them to understand their classmates' contributions. Similarly, they can type their own contributions and have a little more time to formulate their ideas and express them. In face-to-face contexts, words spoken quickly and accents may render understanding difficult. The typed interactions in a MUVE learning activity are slower and free of slurring, challenging accents, and other auditory obstacles. This makes it easier for ESL students as they process the ongoing dialogue contributions of their peers. Anecdotal data from ESL students have consistently suggested that both the frequency of discussion entries and comprehension of the overall discussion are higher in a MUVE setting.

Instructional Note: When a student identifies learning obstacles such as shyness or a language barrier, behavior change can be quantified using transcripts from the students' MUVE learning activities. The instructor (or student) can count the number of times the student speaks via the activity tanscript and can track these data over time. This is one way for a student to make a plan for changing behavior and use data to quantify and track improvement. Both content and quality of contributions to partner or team activities can be monitored. Also, asking shy or passive students to do a self-assessment of their participation can create a more powerful stimulus for change than other forms of direct instructor feedback.

Making Learning Safer for High-Risk Skills

It is not a coincidence that the first learning simulators were for airline pilots. Professionals for whom the consequences of error are serious (a crashed plane, a dead patient) especially benefit from simulation learning. A frequent comment students make about MUVE learning is that "it is a safe place to experiment, to try new behavior and make mistakes without worrying about hurting someone." This is particularly evident in activities that involve one-on-one communication skills. Imagine the importance of students being able to practice end-of-life care discussions before having those conversations with a person who is dying. The MUVE serves as a sandbox, a place to practice and experiment in a setting where the consequences of mistakes are minimized. This provides students with a low-risk environment where they can try out new behavior with less pressure and less risk than doing so in First Life. Students particularly appreciate being able to practice on a MUVE patient before encountering one in a face-to-face clinical situation. Students who practice MUVE job interviews report less pressure and better improvement in their interview skills. The disinhibitory effect enables them to focus better on their actual performance. "I always wanted to be more assertive; this made it easier to practice," one student reported.

Addressing Difficult Student Behaviors: Disrupters, Air Hogs, and Students Who Fly under the Radar

Most instructors have experienced students whose behavior undermines their own learning and sometimes that of their peers as well. Such behavior includes students who overparticipate, those who underparticipate, and those whose participation is disruptive. MUVE learning offers unique opportunities to address and change these behaviors.

One example is the student who overparticipates, the air hog. This student monopolizes discussions, takes up much of the available class air time, and dominates discussion partners. The air hog may be seeking attention, may be bored, or may simply want to dominate the agenda. Whatever the motivation, these students effectively prevent other students from being able to participate equally.

Other students are undercontributors. These students fly under the radar, not doing their share of one-on-one or group work. They do not contribute substantively and rely on the contributions of their partners to complete assigned tasks. Their learning is limited by a passive learning style, underengagement, or failure to meet activity objectives.

A third category are the disrupters. These students do not participate constructively in learning activities but focus instead on actively or passively disrupting learning activities with social interactions, negative comments, or other disruptive behaviors. These three phenomena can occur in one-on-one assignments as well as small group ones, but they are particularly damaging to the effectiveness of one-on-one learning activities. MUVE learning offers a powerful remedy for all three of these learning obstacles.

Talking Story: MUVE Learning as a New Approach to Changing Student Behavior

In one class, several students undermined learning activities with their behavior. All three of the problems described above were illustrated in this group. There were air hogs, there were students flying under the radar, and there were disrupters. A MUVE learning activity offered a new approach to changing these behaviors.

I asked students to do an analysis of transcripts from a series of one-on-one discussions they had completed earlier in the course. The students were asked to analyze the number of times they contributed to the discussion and to report these data as a percentage of the total entries for each discussion they analyzed. Additionally, I asked them to categorize each of their entries. Were their contributions social? Were they content or task specific? Did their contribution move the group forward in the group task or distract from it? The students were asked to complete the same analysis for their activity partner as well. On the basis of these evaluations, students then identified personal goals for improving their one-on-one discussion effectiveness. They were also asked to track progress toward their goals using data from upcoming one-on-one discussions. For the first time in my teaching career, I felt that I had a constructive way to address the behavior of air hogs, disrupters, and students flying under the radar!

The students completed the first round of self-evaluations ("Oops, I was talking 75 percent of the time!"). They made goals ("Since there are two of us, I get only a total of fifteen minutes!). They experimented with new behavior ("My partner is really shy. I need to back off or she will never express herself. Maybe my contribution should be questions to her instead of statements of my own ideas."). Students used transcript data to track, trend, and report on their progress. It became a group game. There were graphs! There were charts! People bragged about their progress from air hog to supportive partner. Another advantage to this approach was that instead of feeling punished or judged, there was a light and often humorous feeling to the process of identifying poor behavior and making a plan to change it. ("Oh NO, there I go again. What an air hog!") When peer review feedback is added to self-evaluations, both based on the objective data an activity transcript provides, this learning activity becomes a powerful vehicle for change.

Slowing Down Communication as a Way of Going Deeper

Typed communication is slower than oral communication. Slowing a discussion down often improves both content and process of the discussion. Participants have more time to think about what has been said and to formulate their own thoughts. There is more time to listen. This MUVE learning advantage is particularly obvious in one-on-one MUVE learning activities.

One of the first things that I noticed when reviewing transcripts from one-on-one MUVE learning activities was that the discussions were more focused and thoughtful than those I had observed in class breakout sessions. Students spent less time in social interactions in the beginning of the discussion; they focused on the assigned task, and key issues were identified more quickly. This made it possible for the learning activity to go deeper faster. Additionally, particularly after students have done analyses of their own discussion contributions, they become more intentional about their own contributions and more sensitive to the contributions of their partners. They begin to work on their partnerships. Comments such as, "Susan, you haven't shared what you think" or "That sounds important, say more about that" are common in MUVE transcripts. In these exchanges, students invite each other to go deeper. The MUVE format increases accountability for interpersonal performance and makes it possible to evaluate it objectively, even tracking improvement over a series of learning activities.

Addressing Obstacles with Learning Activity Design

Strategic use of the MUVE format to overcome some of the obstacles to learning discussed in this chapter is an important part of designing one-on-one MUVE learning activities. This will be addressed later in the chapters that outline the steps for learning activity design.

Reader's Roadmap: Where Are We?

Chapter 7 presented a review of the pedagogical advantages to one-on-one MUVE learning. Chapter 8 will illustrate one-on-on MUVE learning activities through presentation of sample learning activities. This will include a review of the activity's target population, goals, performance outcomes, technical requirements, activity procedures, and evaluation methods.

CHAPTER 8

Sample Learning Activities 4–5

One-on-One MUVE Learning Activities

In this chapter, design features of one-on-one MUVE learning activities are described in detail and specific sample learning activities presented. Descriptions include introduction to the activity, performance outcomes, MUVE setup requirements, activities procedures, and evaluation methods.

This chapter is for you if:

1. You are interested in exploring characteristics of one-on-one MUVE learning activities.

2. You are interested in specific examples of one-on-one MUVE learning activities that could be adapted for your own teaching practice.

Introduction to Sample Learning Activities 4–5: Sample One-on-One Learning Activities

Introduction and Purpose

Any one-on-one professional skill set that is necessary for professional practice can be the basis of a one-on-one MUVE learning activity. Interviewing, communication skills, conflict skills, mediation, and collaboration can all be practiced and objectively evaluated in a one-on-one MUVE learning activity. Getting to know your MUVE activities or exercises or ones designed to develop professional relationships also can be used to identify and quantify behavioral outcomes and to provide the basis for performance improvement plans.

Performance Outcomes

Many possibilities for performance outcomes can be achieved in one-on-one MUVE learning activities. Topical content can be applied, and psychosocial skill sets such as communication, interpersonal leadership, conflict resolution, and emotional intelligence abilities can be practiced, evaluated, and improved in one-on-one MUVE learning activities. Students can practice the skills required for collegial professional and therapeutic relationships. In one-on-one MUVE learning, health care students can practice clinical skills such as patient teaching, counseling, and therapeutic communication interventions as well as teamwork skills such as organization, time management, prioritization, and leadership. Evaluation skills, including self and peer evaluation, can be practiced through a review of learning activity dialogue transcripts.

MUVE Setup

One-on-one MUVE learning activities are low tech. They have no MUVE setup requirements other than identification of the MUVE region where the learning activity will take place. For students new to MUVE learning, it is a good idea to identify a specific region for the learning activity. More experienced students can be encouraged to select a region of their choice. As has been discussed previously, part of the advantage of MUVE learning is contextualizing learning. Some environments support one-on-one interaction better than others. If students select their own locations, it is important to reinforce the importance of selecting a private location where there is a minimal risk of being disturbed.

Activity Procedures

Activity procedures for one-on-one learning activities are simple. Students are assigned a partner and given instructions for the learning activity. If a grading rubric is used for the assignment, it should also be distributed prior to the assignment. After activity completion, students forward the activity transcript to the instructor and complete any evaluations required for the assignment.

The most successful one-on-one MUVE learning activities have specific goals, time limits, and measurable performance outcomes. These should be available to students prior to the activity itself so they can review the instructions and be clear about what is expected of them. It is a good idea to review the learning activity goals and performance expectations in the class setting first, particularly if the class is new to MUVE learning. Students should be held accountable for the time they spend on the learning activity. If the activity is designed for thirty minutes, it should take thirty minutes. Students should not be permitted to use more time to accomplish the goal of the activity. An important performance outcome is that the activity be completed within the specified period of time.

Evaluation

The evaluation of one-on-one MUVE learning activity is based on specific learning objectives and performance outcomes the instructor has identified for the activity. Both content material and behavioral tasks can be the focus of the activity. For example, if the learning activity requires a patient interview that focuses on a patient history, an evaluation matrix of the learning activity could include all items the instructor requires to be included in the history. Interpersonal skills can also be effectively practiced. Such an activity could focus on demonstration of skills required for a therapeutic or professional collegial relationship. For all these skills, a self-evaluation might be appropriate in which students identify what went well during the assignment and what they would like to do differently in the future. Evaluation in this case could be specific to behavior of students during the interview. In short, evaluation of one-on-one MUVE learning activities will be dependent on the learning activity performance outcomes and specific to the goals of the learning activity. Peer evaluations added to a self-evaluation requirement strengthen the evaluation process. If portfolio evaluation is used, transcripts for learning activities in MUVE can be added to portfolio documentation, in addition to the completed evaluation matrix for the activity.

Evaluation Grid for Tracking Individual Learning Activity Effectiveness over Time

MUVE learning activity: _____   Semester: _____   Year: _____

Criteria	Semester 1	Semester 2	Semester 3	Semester 4	Semester 5	Semester Average
Percentage of students who met 100 percent of learning objectives for the semester						
Percentage of students who met > 80 percent of learning objectives for the semester						
Percentage of students who met > 70 percent of learning objectives for the semester						
Percentage of students who met < 70 percent learning objectives for the semester						
Percentage of groups that met small group learning objectives						

Summative and Formative Assessment Procedures
for One-on-One MUVE Learning Activities

Use of transcripts for learning activity and course evaluation is a great benefit for instructors. Not only can students receive objective feedback on the basis of their actual performance, but also instructors can track total class performance on individual learning activities and the effectiveness of the MUVE activities across the semester. From semester to semester, the instructor can also track effectiveness of the activity itself as it is modified and improved. From an instructor perspective, this is a huge pedagogical advantage. It takes very few minutes to scan a thirty-minute learning activity and to grade both individual and group performance. The instructor can keep group data from semester to semester to quantify the effectiveness of MUVE learning.

Instructional Note: It is a good idea to include requirements for peer review in the total points for an assignment. The student can receive points for both completing a peer review for another student and incorporating a peer review into their own performance improvement plan. Just grading a peer as "good" is not enough. Students should be required to either complete quantitative evaluations (Likert scales) and/or describe specifically what was good. An instructor can also require that peer feedback be incorporated into the student's performance improvement plan. This process enhances the learning activity by including performance improvement skills among the others included in the activity. Instructor feedback on student peer feedback is also an important part of the process.

Portfolio Evaluation

If a course is using portfolio evaluation, the transcript for each learning activity, the completed grading matrix, and the self, peer, and instructor evaluations can all be included as data in students' course portfolios. If students are tracking their performance over time, data can be added to a performance tracking summary. (See Appendix 5 for an example.)

Examples of One-on-One MUVE Learning Activities

There are limitless opportunities for one-on-one MUVE learning activities. The following are examples of specific learning activities that were used with nursing students. The first, Introduction to Patient Interviewing, is designed for undergraduate nurses early in their first semester; the second is for advanced practice nurses at the graduate level. For each learning activity, the following are included: an introduction to the activity, a brief description of the activity goals, the target learner population, performance outcomes, setup requirements, procedural steps for the activity, and activity evaluation methods.

Sample Learning Activity 4: Interviewing a Patient

Introduction and Purpose

This is a MUVE learning activity for entry-level clinical students who are required to be able to demonstrate basic patient interviewing skills. For this activity, students work in pairs. One student is assigned the role of interviewer and the other is assigned the role of patient. The thirty-minute interview covers the main elements of a patient interview as outlined by the instructor in an activity grading matrix. This activity is designed to give students an opportunity to demonstrate skills required for a patient interview. The interviewer's goal is to demonstrate all required elements of the patient interview. The patient's goal is to use a prepared case study to act out a patient case study during the interview. The interviewer receives a grade for the quality of the interview. The patient's grade is based on the quality of the case study.

Target Population

Target students for this activity are clinical practice students who have completed a didactic presentation that covers required elements for a patient interview. This learning activity is ideal for first-year nursing students after they have completed classes that cover a patient interview for health history and history of symptoms. This is the type of learning activity that is traditionally videotaped by the instructor for review and critique, which is extremely time-consuming. When the activity is done in a MUVE, it is easier to evaluate and practical for use multiple times throughout a semester.

Performance Outcomes

At the end of the forty-five- to sixty-minute learning activity, students will have completed the following:

1. A detailed health history and history of the presenting illness as outlined in the class and according to a grading matrix that identifies all items that should be covered.

2. Demonstration of elements of therapeutic communication (specific elements can be identified in the grading matrix and may include communication techniques such as active listening, mirroring, reflecting).

MUVE Setup

1. A specific MUVE clinical location is identified for the MUVE learning activity. In Second Life®, a hospital such as Second Health Hospital, a clinic, or a nurse practitioner office can be used. Students should not be permitted to do this activity in a social environment. They should be reminded of the professional requirements of their learning activities, patient privacy, protection of health care data, and support of a therapeutic relationship.

2. Students should be assigned partners. The pairs of students arrange a time to meet to complete the learning activity. This activity is more effective if students do not pick their friends as partners. Social relationships between friends can be an obstacle to performance of therapeutic relationship skills. This is a key element to the development of therapeutic relationships.

Activity Procedures

1. One student is assigned to be the interviewer. His or her partner acts in the patient role. This activity is most effective if new pairs are formed for each interview, alternating roles each time the assignment is done. Included in the grading matrix can be points allocated for serving as the patient.

2. The student acting in the patient role will use a case study distributed only to the students acting in the patient role. They are encouraged to improvise and act out the role they are playing. Two case studies should be prepared for this assignment so that no student interacts twice with the same patient case study.

3. The interviewer will complete a history and review of systems and symptom history with the patient, using the "History and Physical" form provided by the instructor.

4. At the end of the interview, the interviewer will copy the chat transcript and forward it to his or her partner for peer review. Self and peer evaluations can use the grading matrix for the assignment. Additional comments/suggestions (positive feedback and suggestions for improvements) can be added.

5. The entire evaluation packet is then attached to the activity transcript and forwarded to the instructor. The instructor adds an evaluation,

feedback, and suggestions and returns the packet to students with final grading.

6. The instructor completes summative and formative evaluation for the activity.

Evaluation

1. Using the grading matrix, both the student and his or her peer complete an evaluation of the interviewer and forward it along with a copy of the transcript to the instructor. Both evaluations can include the actual grade from the matrix, as well as identified areas of strength and weakness and suggestions for improvement.

2. The total grade for the assignment includes points allocated for completion within the time identified for the assignment, completion of a peer review for their partners, and interpersonal communication/therapeutic relationship skills.

3. Portfolio: If a portfolio is being used for course assessment, the transcript of the learning activity and the self, peer, and instructor evaluations can be included.

Sample Learning Activity 5: A Nurse Practitioner Clinic

Introduction and Purpose

In this learning activity, a pair of nurse practitioner students demonstrate evaluation and care planning for a patient with a specific disease (identified by the instructor). The student acting as the patient creates a typical case study of a patient with the assigned pathology. The other student acts in the role of nurse practitioner. The purpose of the activity is for students to use the role of nurse practitioner to practice interviewing, assessment, and care planning for a patient with a specific disease. In the role of patient, students formulate a case study that profiles typical presentation of the disease that is the focus of the activity.

The student acting as the nurse practitioner is evaluated on ability to perform a complete assessment of the patient and formulate differential diagnoses, a final diagnosis, and a plan of care that includes a teaching plan. Students in the role of the patient are evaluated on their presentation of a typical, comprehensive, coherent, and plausible patient. Their assignment will include a plan of care for the patient and a teaching plan.

Target Population

This assignment is ideal for novice nurse practitioner students who have completed basic courses in the curriculum and who are preparing for clinical experiences.

Performance Outcomes

1. In the history and physical exam, the student in the nurse practitioner role will be expected to demonstrate knowledge of risk factors, lab values, and physical findings that are characteristic of the pathology focus for the learning activity.

2. In the formulation of the case study, the student in the patient role will be expected to demonstrate knowledge of risk factors, differential, lab values, and physical findings that are characteristic of the pathology focus for the learning activity.

3. In both roles, students are expected to be able to utilize the learning transcript to formulate differential diagnoses, a final diagnosis, a treatment plan, and a patient education plan for the pathology that is the focus of the learning activity.

MUVE Setup

Students should be directed to a MUVE region that provides a clinical environment such as a professional office, hospital clinical unit, or community clinic. Second Health Hospital or other hospitals in Second Life® are often good locations. Students will be assigned roles for this assignment, half in the role of nurse practitioner and the other half in the role of patient. Both groups will be told the disease focus for the assignment.

Activity Procedures

1. The instructor assigns pairs and roles for the assignment and identifies the target disease pathology for the assignment.

2. Students in the role of patient formulate a case study for a patient with the disease identified in the assignment. The goal of the case study is to present a typical case presentation, including risk factors, psychosocial issues, lab values, diagnostic test findings, and so on. In acting out this case study, patients provide their partner with the interview,

diagnostic, and physical findings data needed to make a plan of care for the patient. This involves some creativity. If a nurse practitioner says, "I am palpating your pulses now," the patient should respond with clinical data: "They are bilateral +4 and bounding." The nurse practitioner can ask, "Do you have any abnormal lab values or diagnostic test findings?" The patient can respond with a report of relevant data: "The CT scan was negative." The assignment grade for students in the patient role is based on the case study formulation, its presentation, and the final care and teaching plans.

3. The nurse practitioner's assignment is to interview the patient in the simulated nurse practitioner's clinic office. The grade is based on their interview of the patient, the differential and final diagnoses, and the final care and teaching plan.

4. Both participants will meet inworld at an agreed-upon time. They will complete the interview within sixty minutes.

5. After the interview, both students review the transcript and create both a plan of care and a teaching plan for the patient.

   Instructional Note: If, upon reviewing the transcript, either student identifies mistakes, omissions, or things he or she would do differently, these items can be addressed in the final plan of care typed in red. As this reflects self-assessment and ongoing learning, I typically give at least partial credit for these additions.

6. Using the grading grid for the assignment, the student acting in the role of the nurse practitioner completes a self-evaluation of the interview, including a final grade and identification of areas of strength and those with a need for improvement. The student who acted in the role of patient completes a peer evaluation of the nurse practitioner's performance in the activity.

Evaluation

The plans of care, teaching plans, and both participants' evaluations are submitted with the interview transcript to the instructor for final evaluation, grading, and feedback. If the course includes portfolio evaluation, a copy of the transcript, the grading matrix, and the peer evaluation are included in the portfolio. A sample template for use in evaluating the generic parts of this assignment can be found in Appendix 2.

Instructional Note: This assignment involves a wide range of skills and knowledge sets. It requires preparation and follow-up for both participants.

Over the course of a semester, students should alternate between the patient and nurse practitioner roles. One way to accomplish this is to use a matrix of assignment pairs. The assignment matrix enables students to be paired with a different student every week. By the end of the semester, each student will have been in the roles of both nurse practitioner with each classmate at least once and patient for each classmate as well. Students alternate roles each week so they are patient and nurse practitioner an equal number of times.

A third sample of an effective one-on-one learning activity, Mock Job Interview, is located in Appendix 3. In this activity, nurses at all levels can practice job interview skills, get feedback, make plans for skill improvement, and implement these plans in repeated MUVE practice interviews.

Tools to Use: How to Chat and Copy a Second Life® Learning Activity Transcript

To copy the learning activity dialogue from a chat box:

1. Along the bottom of the Second Life® viewer, there appears a row of icons. The farthest one to the left is Chat and appears next to a chat balloon icon. Click on the icon.

2. A chat box appears on the Second Life® viewer. To make an entry into the chat box, type your entry in the blank chat box and hit enter.

3. This enters a comment into the ongoing discussion. Both the name of the person making the entry and the time (Second Life® clock time) accompany the entry. Any other avatar within thirty (inworld) feet of you will see the entry in the chat box on their Second Life® viewer and can reply to you.

4. Each discussion entry is preceded with a time stamp and the name of the person who made the comment.

5. When the chat box is used in a one-on-one or small group learning activity, each entry is added to the chat box. Only the most recent three or four are visible in the chat box, but if you scroll up, you will find the entire discussion.

6. Once the discussion or learning activity is completed, any participant can highlight the entire chat from the chat box and paste it into a Word file on their computer. This file constitutes a written transcript of the learning activity and can be used as documentation of the event, for use in self-evaluation, peer evaluation, or for instructor evaluation of student performance individually and/or as groups. Additionally, the

transcripts can be used to evaluate group process or interpersonal/ group dynamics. Students also sometimes keep the transcripts as notes for the content that was covered during the learning activity.

Reader's Roadmap: Where Are We?

This completes the introduction of MUVE one-on-one learning activities. Chapter 9 will present the pedagogical benefits of small group learning, and Chapter 10 will review the design elements for and examples of small group MUVE learning activities.

CHAPTER 9

Pedagogical Benefits of MUVE
Small Group Learning Activities

This chapter reviews the pedagogical benefits of MUVE small group learning activities, such as accountability for small group participation, quantification of small group dynamics, and changing dysfunctional group behavior.

This chapter is for you if:

1. You are interested in MUVE small group learning activities.

2. You are planning a MUVE small group learning activity.

Pedagogical Benefits of MUVE Small Group Learning

Many of the pedagogical benefits offered by one-on-one MUVE learning activities also apply to MUVE small group learning. Small group MUVE learning is situated, self-directed, and independent with a high degree of objective self, peer, and group evaluation using activity transcript analysis. In addition, several teaching and learning benefits are specific to MUVE small group learning.

Group Participation Accountability

Transcript analysis of small group learning activities affords a high degree of accountability for members' contribution to both the team task and group process performance. Using a learning activity analysis matrix and the activity transcript, students can perform self, peer, and group evaluations. These include analysis of skills related to group task achievement as well as individual and teamwork skills. Both activity grades and suggestions for improvement can be based on objective data. This level of objectivity and data-driven feedback is only possible in traditional face-to-face small group activities if they are video recorded, a resource-intensive process that is rarely practical. Even in simulation laboratories with video capability, review of video is not only time-consuming but also cumbersome.

Using transcript analysis to evaluate MUVE learning activities can also assist the course instructor with intervention in small group problems that are difficult to address in face-to-face learning activities. One such problem that creates significant student dissatisfaction in small group work is fair evaluation of the quality and quantity of individual members' contribution to face-to-face small group assignments. Students often complain of inequality in both quality and quantity of group members' contributions. Some group members dominate the group while others habitually undercontribute. Still other group members may disrupt or otherwise undermine group productivity. When this kind of inequity in contributions to group work occurs, group performance and morale are both seriously affected.

Unless a face-to-face small group activity is videotaped, there is no way for an instructor to evaluate the quality of each student's group contributions. It is similarly difficult to identify and address inequality in group participation. In addition, when less formal evaluation methods are used, important prosocial group behaviors such as group leadership, constructive feedback, affirmation, mediation, or conflict resolution may not be identified. Use of transcript analysis in the evaluation process makes this possible.

When a MUVE small group activity transcript is used for self-evaluation, students can easily identify their own under- or overparticipation. Disruptive behavior is obvious. Data provided from activity transcripts are objective and can provide the basis for peer and instructor feedback as well as plans for performance improvement. When students know that transcript analysis is part of every group discussion, they participate more consistently and at a higher level. Thus, one significant pedagogical benefit of MUVE small group learning is the degree to which the volume, quality, and actual work of small group membership can be objectively evaluated. Student accountability becomes the rule, not the exception, and assignment grading is data driven, reflecting actual individual performance.

Group Dynamics

When analysis of a MUVE small group discussion transcript is a routine part of a small group learning activity, there is greater accountability for group dynamics. Group phenomena that obstruct effective learning, such as interpersonal conflict, subgrouping, or collusion with underperformance, are easy to identify in the activity transcript. On the basis of the transcript data, behavior can be identified and goals set for student behavior change. The objectivity of this process reduces what can potentially be an emotionally charged problem. A teachable moment occurs when students review the transcript data themselves and the instructor offers theory and content specific to dysfunctional group dynamics. Students can evaluate their own performance against specific criteria. The instructor can then offer suggestions for performance improvement. The group's own ongoing self-evaluations become the foundation for continuing improvement and accountability.

Inexperienced small groups often have difficulty identifying causes of group dysfunction. They may lack either knowledge to articulate and problem solve or the interpersonal skills to confront problems in the group. They usually simply report that the group is not working. Individual group members may express dissatisfaction to the instructor or each other. In this case, group work products are often negatively affected. Using transcript evaluation and analysis can help a group identify causes of group dysfunction. This improves not only group satisfaction but also group work products. In addition, the group has an opportunity to learn invaluable lessons about group dynamics and constructive conflict resolution.

In situations in which the group knows perfectly well what is wrong with the group (one person dominates or does all the work, underparticipation is not confronted, or there is disruptive behavior), data from analysis of learning activity transcripts can be used to improve group performance. The group can use transcript data to identify problems, plan for solutions, and evaluate the effectiveness of their plan. Using this evaluation method, the group develops skills for both evaluating and improving team performance. As the transcripts are evaluated over time, the small group has the opportunity to track their group performance improvement. The instructor's role is to support this performance evaluation and improvement process, as well as to guide students with theory and specific skill guidance.

Talking Story: Changing Group Behavior

Leaving class one day, I trailed behind a group of class members leaving our classroom. One of them was obviously blowing off steam. "I just hate small group. It is always the same. I do all the work or it just doesn't get done." One of her friends nodded and offered, "Just confront the other people and tell them they have to do their part." Her friend snorted and answered, "Right, except that doing that and holding their feet to the fire is more work than just doing it myself. At least I know the group will get a high grade if I do most of the work."

I have heard complaints like this many times before. Occasionally, a group member such as this will meet with me and complain that others are not doing their work. Often, they do not perceive that their own overfunctioning may be related to the underfunctioning of others. Students' perceptions that making others do their work increases their own work or that leaving the group to flounder results in a poor grade are hard to dispute. I decided to try an experiment. I changed the planned small group MUVE learning activity. It was to have been optional, but instead I made it mandatory for the whole class. This meant adding MUVE orientation to my class plan and a bit of juggling and finessing, but I thought it would be worth it. I told the members of the class who had not participated in the previous voluntary MUVE activities, "You only have to do it this once."

The next discussion group included a transcript analysis of the MUVE learning activity. Because the class focus was research, I turned it into a data analysis project. We talked in class prior to the assignment about qualitative and quantitative data and the importance of analyzing both. I offered an illustration of the way that both quantitative and qualitative data could be used to evaluate small group teamwork. Students were assigned a small group discussion in which they discussed a specific ethical topic. After the assignment, each student analyzed both his or her contributions to the group and those for each group participant. Each student received points for frequency and quality of contributions, as well as gems (contributions of particularly high value). Not every group loved it, but every group improved. Patterns of under- and overperformance were clear. Groups were clearly confronted with opportunities to improve team performance. The class learned to hold all team members objectively accountable for team tasks. Overall, small group participation improved once students knew that there was an objective way to evaluate their performance.

Leadership Development

MUVE learning offers a unique opportunity for students to practice small group leadership skills, even if leadership is not the focus of the class. MUVE discussion groups, clinical rounds, or other MUVE small group activities give students a chance to practice leadership skills. A MUVE learning activity offers students a way to improve leadership skills through specific feedback from both peers and the course instructor. Courses that focus on leadership development and group leadership responsibilities can be included in learning activity requirements. In other classes, extra credit can be offered for students who volunteer to provide small group leadership. The MUVE learning activity transcript can be used for evaluation of leadership performance, not only in students' self-evaluations but also through feedback from peers and the course instructor. Such evaluations are based on the performance requirements of the individual MUVE learning activity and can be quantified through the assignment grading rubric.

Grading Equity

Grading of traditional small group activities is often a sore subject for students doing small group projects. In groups in which one or more students under-participate, the other students have to contribute more work toward the total group grade. This contribution inequity constitutes an unfairness that is difficult for students to confront among themselves and impossible for faculty to confront without specific data. Usually, all students from such a group get the same grade for the group assignment. Everyone involved, including the instructor, is usually aware of the unfairness of this system but lack the data to make it more equitable.

If small group planning meetings are in themselves MUVE activities, transcript data and subsequent work product evaluation can provide the basis for grading that is objective and specific to each group member. Grade the planning sessions! What a novel idea! If the instructor chooses, transcript data can be used to determine individual as well as group grades for group project planning and execution. This can result in significant improvement in students' attitudes toward small group work. The students who typically do most of the work feel that it is more fair. Students who typically underparticipate are held accountable with objective data. The group planning transcripts can be used to keep a record of students' assignments, follow-up, and performance. This effectively creates "minutes" of the group meeting, for which group members are held accountable.

Economy and Quality of Learning

Small group MUVE learning activities take less time than face-to-face groups. When small groups meet face-to-face in class, time is lost physically moving from the classroom to the small group meeting location. More time is expended as the group settles down to the task; gets started; moves through socially awkward moments, distractions, and disruptions; and then finally focuses on task completion. Frequently, only half of the allotted time for small group learning is productive, task-focused interaction. If small groups meet in one place (for example, in the classroom), there is little privacy, and the noise of so many people talking at once can interfere with group communication. This is not the case in a MUVE small group activity. In a MUVE learning activity, learning takes place in an undistracting and relatively private environment. Because the students are aware there is a transcript of the activity, the learning activity starts and focuses very quickly. Typically, the meeting objectives are met through a satisfying and enriching process. When students know there is a transcript of the discussion, they get the work done! When they do not, the transcript provides clear evidence of this for grading purposes.

MUVE learning activities such as discussion groups can be offered as an option in lieu of class time. In classes where I do this, the small group discussion portion of the class happens in the last hour of class. Students have the option of staying for the face-to-face discussion group. Students who choose the MUVE discussion option leave class as the face-to-face discussions begin, after scheduling a meeting time for their MUVE discussion group. Group members can be at home, in the student lounge, or in the school library. Often, busy students prefer such discussions to be in the evening, on weekends, or early in the morning. When surveyed, even students who do not particularly like MUVE learning agree that such discussion groups are highly convenient, are efficient, and provide a high-quality learning experience. There is a learning efficiency and effectiveness offered in this kind of learning that supports good use of the resources of time and energy for students.

Talking Story: Not for Every Student?

A student in one of my classes was one of those brilliant students who inspires both their peers and their teachers with the depth and passion of their learning. I was disappointed when this student chose not to participate in optional MUVE small groups, choosing the face-to-face option instead. I kept saying, "Try it! I think you are going to love it." He consistently answered, "Nursing is face-to-face and that is how I prefer to learn." But after hearing his peers rave about their MUVE groups, he tried one. I still have the lengthy e-mail he sent me afterward. He discussed at length the differences he saw, the depth of the learning, the density of the activity, its economy, the energy it generated, what a good thing it was for nursing, and how much fun it was. He concluded by saying, "I get it now. I totally get what you are doing with the MUVE activities, but I still prefer learning face-to-face." MUVE learning, even when its advantages are appreciated by students, may still not be their preferred way to learn.

General Description of Small Group MUVE Learning Activities

Introduction and Purpose

Small group MUVE learning activities are diverse and can be used to address a wide range of performance outcomes. They can be very simple activities or quite complex. They can be used to focus on specific course content or engage group process outcomes.

Group process and group dynamics such as collaboration can be evaluated easily using the MUVE transcript. This means that group evaluation skills such as performance evaluation and group processes such as collaboration, problem solving, or conflict management can be easily evaluated. Small group MUVE learning thus has the potential for a higher degree of complexity than solo or one-on-one MUVE learning.

Target Population

MUVE small group activities are appropriate for a wide range of learners. They are highly effective for undergraduate, graduate, and doctoral-level students. The number of participants can affect learning effectiveness. For most MUVE small group activities, there should be approximately six participants. Fewer than four can create a less effective group dynamic, as there is more pressure on each participant. With greater than six participants, it can be difficult for all individuals to participate sufficiently.

Performance Outcomes

Performance outcomes for small group MUVE learning activities can include demonstration of topical content application, interpersonal skills, emotional intelligence abilities, evaluation skills (self, peer, and group evaluation skills), collegial and interdisciplinary relationship skills, clinical skills such as interviewing, development and maintenance of therapeutic relationships, one-on-one teaching, patient counseling, therapeutic communication interventions, and teamwork skills such as task organization, time management, and task prioritization.

MUVE Setup

Small group MUVE learning activities require more detailed planning than solo and one-on-one MUVE activities do. It is recommended that novice MUVE instructors begin with relatively simple MUVE activities such as discussion groups, moving to more complex activities after basic instructional MUVE skills are well established.

Activity Procedures

The success of a group MUVE learning activity depends on a clear set of procedural steps for the activity. The instructor should outline steps for the activity prior to beginning student orientation to the activity. More complex MUVE small group activities may involve the addition of more sophisticated instructor MUVE skills. For example, an instructor may choose to manage several avatars at once during a learning activity. In the Second Life® exam described in Chapter 2, the instructor uses four to five different avatars. ("See Tools to Use: How to Manage Two Avatars at One Time" in Chapter 11.)

Evaluation of Small Group Activities in MUVE

An evaluation matrix for a small group MUVE learning activity focuses on objectives for the learning activity. These may include course content, communication skills, and team skills. All group participants can be evaluated on one grading matrix. The matrix can include criteria for each individual's performance as well as group performance outcomes. Summative activity data can also be included on the same matrix. Because MUVE small group activities involve more peers and an entire group to evaluate, both the sophistication and volume of evaluation possible with small group MUVE learning activities are greater than with other MUVE learning forms.

Portfolio Evaluation

If portfolio evaluation is used, transcripts for small group MUVE learning activities may be added to the students' portfolios. Self, peer, and summary instructor evaluations may also be included. This opportunity for 360-degree evaluation using the objective data from the MUVE small group learning activity transcript is unique and valuable. Because small group MUVE learning activities are typically complex, summative and formative evaluation of the instructional activity itself is an important part of the evaluation process. This provides a means for instructors to both track instructional performance improvement and improve the learning activities themselves.

Reader's Roadmap: Where Are We?

This chapter has reviewed and described the pedagogical benefits of small group MUVE learning activities. Chapters 10–12 will present detailed descriptions of basic, advanced, and complex MUVE small group learning activities.

CHAPTER 10

Sample Learning Activities 6–8

Ethics, Genetics, and Disability Small Group Activities

This chapter illustrates the pedagogical benefits of MUVE small group discussions described in Chapter 9 by presenting three in-depth illustrations of basic-level small group MUVE learning activities: Ethics, Genetics, and Disabilities Discussion Groups. Descriptions of these activities will include the following: an introduction to the activity, performance outcomes, MUVE setup requirements, activity procedures, and evaluation methods.

This chapter is for you if:

1. You are interested MUVE small group learning activities.

2. You are planning your first MUVE small group learning activity.

3. You are interested in the format of a simple topical discussion group.

Sample Learning Activity 6: Ethics Discussion Group

Introduction and Purpose

In this activity, students apply ethics course work in a small group setting in a MUVE. The purpose of this learning activity is to engage undergraduate students in small group discussions in which they apply ethics concepts reviewed in class to specific ethical issues.

Target Population

The activity works best when there are five to six students in each discussion group. The assignment is most successful when a student is assigned to lead the group discussion. One way to orient students to group leadership is to provide all students with a list of expectations for group leadership. The course instructor may choose to lead the first discussion group, to provide role modeling.

Performance Outcomes

At the end of each thirty-minute ethics discussion group, participants will have demonstrated the following (the asterisk refers to objectives for the designated group leader alone):

1. Identification of ethical principles (autonomy, fidelity, beneficence, nonmaleficence, paternalism) illustrated in the ethical dilemma under discussion.

2. Identification of the ethical principle that most describes their own personal view of the ethical dilemma under discussion.

3. Approximately equal contributions from all participants.

4. At least one instance of feedback to a peer during the discussion (agreeing, disagreeing, affirming, requesting an expansion of or query about their statement, etc.).

5. Participation in formulation of a consensus statement for the questions posed in the discussion group assignments.

*6. The group leader will welcome students, start the group on time, state the group task, facilitate the group discussion, assist the group with staying on task, serve as timekeeper, end the discussion on time, and send the discussion transcript to participants and the course instructor after the activity is completed.

Instructional Note: To achieve full credit points for this activity, each student is expected to contribute in both volume and quality of input and to respond to another group member at least once. The group as a whole is expected to complete the assigned task within the time allotted.

MUVE Setup

There are no particular setup requirements for the Ethics Discussion Group. The class should receive orientation to the activity in writing and in class so any questions about the activity can be answered prior to the day of the activity. The location for the learning activity can either be assigned by the instructor or selected by the group leader. The location of the learning activity should be selected on the basis of its privacy and other esthetic criteria. For example, a beautiful and secluded environment that appears comfortable may help participants feel relaxed and comfortable with sharing difficult ideas.

Activity Procedures

1. Group signup: The instructor may assign discussion groups or the class may form groups independently. For logistical ease, it is usually best to have students pick their own group to participate in. Group members who know each other's schedule often find it easier to agree on meeting times for the activity. It works well to either assign leaders or to offer extra credit for students willing to be group leaders. In either case, group leaders post the time, date, and location of the MUVE learning activity they are leading. Students can then sign up with them directly. This can be done in class if the course meets in person or online in an online discussion thread in an online course.

2. Discussion group membership: Small MUVE discussion groups work best with six participants (one leader, five participants). A seventh participant makes the group cumbersome, and it often takes the group longer to complete group tasks. (I typically exercise some flexibility here depending on class size.) Eight or more students are not recommended for this activity. Groups of fewer than four participants are not recommended.

3. The instructor e-mails group leaders the topic for group discussion and the leadership evaluation matrix so that leaders are clear what is expected of them. The group members are sent a description of the discussion assignment and the assignment grading matrix.

4. The group meets in the MUVE region they have selected and the discussion is completed within the specified time period. Note: individuals who arrive late have points deducted, and it is recommended that they not receive credit for the assignment if they are more than a few minutes late. Because this assignment is relatively short and the flow of discussion easily disrupted, it is essential that all group members are on time for the assignment.

5. The small group leader copies the discussion transcript and mails it to all group members and the course instructor.

6. Depending on the assignment evaluation plan, individual, peer, and/or group evaluations are completed by the students and group leaders.

7. Grades and feedback are distributed to groups, individual members, and the group leader.

8. The instructor completes formative and summative evaluation for the learning activity, including quantifiable student performance data and anecdotal data from student feedback and comments.

Evaluation

Formative and summative evaluation is completed by the instructor. Average percentages for student grades, percentages of individuals who met the assignment objectives, and performance scores for the class as a whole can be summarized to track individual, class, and learning activity performance. If a portfolio evaluation is used for the class, copies of the activity transcript, completed grading matrices, areas of strengths and opportunities for improvement, and the self, peer, and group evaluations can all become elements of the portfolio. (See Appendixes 6–9 for samples of student self, peer, and group evaluation matrices, as well as instructor summary forms.)

Instructional Notes: The designation of a group leader is essential for the success of this activity. MUVE discussion groups without leaders often struggle with task completion and group process. An assigned group leader supports a better learning activity and development of leadership skills. It also enables the instructor to focus primarily on evaluation and feedback for the activity.

For classes that meet in person, MUVE learning activities can be done in lieu of class time. If the class is mandatory, class time can be shortened. When offering a MUVE alternative to an in-class assignment such as a discussion group, the last forty-five to sixty minutes of class can be devoted to the discussion group, and students doing the MUVE activity can leave the class. If the assignment is mandatory for all students, the instructor has the option of shortening class accordingly.

Sample Learning Activity 7: Genetics Discussion Group

Introduction and Purpose

The goal of this learning activity is student application of knowledge about family genetic charts to discussion of genetic disease transmission. This will include calculation of disease probability for diseases associated with dominant or recessive gene inheritance and application of course genetics content to a discussion of specific family case studies.

Target Population

This activity is particularly good for small group discussions. At the undergraduate level, the activity should be led by an instructor. Graduate students can do this activity independently in small groups.

Performance Outcomes

Upon completion of a thirty-minute learning activity, students will have:

1. Evaluated three family genetic charts, identifying and discussing the modes of transmission for each of the charts.

2. Given examples of diseases that are represented by the type of genetic abnormality transmission for each chart evaluated.

3. Demonstrated effective participation in the group discussion, including substantive contributions as well as feedback to peers.

MUVE Setup

The only setup requirement is the identification of a location on Genome Island in Second Life® that is suitable for a small group discussion. The outdoor lounge at the laboratory is ideal.

Activity Procedures

1. Students will be oriented to the small group activity and assigned a small group, which will agree on a date and time to meet inworld.

2. The small group will meet at the Genome Island landing area and proceed to the lounge platform of the laboratory structure (near the landing area).

3. For thirty minutes, students will click on one of the family genetic charts that hover over the lounge area. The group will discuss the genetic transmission it represents, as well as the diseases that are transmitted in that manner. Instructors can highlight specific issues related to the type of transmission and lead a discussion of specific diseases.

4. At the end of the discussion period, students copy the discussion transcript and send it to the instructor, along with sketches of each chart that was discussed and their individual, peer, and/or group evaluation.

Evaluation

Evaluation of this learning activity will depend on the instructor's criteria for each chart the group discusses. Points are also awarded based on student contributions to the group activity as well as their feedback to peers during the activity. A sample grading matrix is included in Appendix 10.

Sample Learning Activity 8: Disabilities Discussion Group

Introduction and Purpose

In this learning activity, a small group of students will explore Second Life®'s Virtual Ability Island to introduce a range of topics related to caring for individuals with disabilities.

Target Population

This activity is particularly good for small groups of undergraduate students, who can build on this treasure hunt with later group discussions on a wide variety of topics involving caring for people with disabilities. This learning activity does not require an assigned leader, but it is required that the group stay together (the group should not divide up to find the items). This can be evaluated using the activity transcript, which is required for learning activity evaluation.

Performance Outcomes

Upon completion of a thirty-minute learning activity, students will have worked together as a group to locate resources on the island that will help them demonstrate the following:

1. Description of four kinds of access barriers for people with physical disabilities.

2. Identification of a definition and description of both neurological and cognitive disabilities.

3. Identification of a definition and description of auditory and speech disabilities, as well as two strategies for working with each.

4. Discussion of issues related to the public image of people with disabilities and identification of terms that can be used to describe those who are disabled.

5. Evaluation of the learning activity transcript of the learning activity and documentation of their own answers to the questions posed by the activity.

MUVE Setup

None.

Activity Procedures

1. Students will be oriented to the small group activity and assigned a small group. The group will agree on a date and time to meet in Second Life®.

2. The small group will meet at the Virtual Ability Island landing area and proceed to the series of connected informational platforms that present a number of issues related to a variety of types of disability.

3. For thirty minutes, students will explore each of the platforms together, reading and reviewing the presentation material to answer the assignment questions.

4. At the end of the discussion period, students will copy the discussion transcript and send it to the instructor, along with answers to the assignment questions and summaries of individual, peer, and/or group evaluations.

Evaluation

Evaluation of this learning activity will depend on the instructor's evaluation of the extent to which each group met the learning activities. For a sample of a grading matrix that can be used, see Appendix 11.

Reader's Roadmap: Where Are We?

Part II concludes with Chapters 11 and 12, which present two complex small group MUVE learning activities. The Clinical Rounds learning activity in Chapter 11 illustrates a MUVE learning activity with complex content and structure. The Building Small Group Consensus Skills learning activity in Chapter 12 focuses on complex group dynamics and team-building competencies.

CHAPTER 11

Sample Learning Activity 9 (Complex Small Group MUVE Learning Activity)

Clinical Rounds

The purpose of this chapter is to illustrate a complex MUVE small group learning activity. This illustration demonstrates that a MUVE learning activity can offer effective learning and achieve learning outcomes that are difficult to achieve using traditional methodologies.

This chapter is for you if:

1. You are interested in designing a complex MUVE learning activity.

2. You are interested in a form of clinical simulation that offers the pedagogical advantages of MUVE learning.

Sample Learning Activity 9: Clinical Rounds

Introduction and Purpose

MUVE learning is a form of simulation learning. In any clinical simulation, students are emerged in a clinical scenario, learning together in an environment similar to ones in which they will practice in the future. "Clinical rounds" is a MUVE simulation in which health care students, guided by a group activity leader, do clinical rounds on a patient who has a disease the students are studying in class.

The purpose of this activity is to explore specific disease pathologies by interviewing patients who have the disease. A small group of health care students spend thirty minutes in a MUVE hospital reviewing a specific disease, briefly talking with a patient who has the disease that is the focus of the learning activity, and then discussing as a small group the care planning and clinical management appropriate for the patient. Although designed originally for nursing students, this activity would work well for medical students, respiratory therapists, or students from other health care disciplines.

Target Population

This activity is effective for both undergraduate- and graduate-level health care students. For novice practitioners or undergraduate students, this exercise is typically led by the course instructor. The "patient" is either a teaching assistant or the instructor, who in this instance would be "controlling" two avatars at once, one as the learning activity leader and the other as the patient. For graduate students or those in advanced practice courses (nurse practitioners, clinical nurse specialists, medical students), the learning activity can be designed so that students take turns assuming both activity leader and patient roles. Activity leaders can be graded according to a grading rubric specific to clinical rounds. Students acting in the role of patient can be graded according to their ability to design and execute a representative case study for the disease being discussed.

Performance Outcomes

By the end of the thirty-minute clinical rounds learning activity, participants will have:

1. Met on time at the MUVE region chosen for the learning activity.

2. As a group, reviewed essential information about the pathology focus for the learning activity

3. Identified disease specific issues that should be raised with the patient (steps 1 through 3 take ten minutes).

4. Briefly discussed the patient's condition with the patient, identifying his or her priority issues and concerns.

5. Asked the patient a few questions related to his or her condition, coping, knowledge, and so on (steps 4 and 5 take ten minutes).

6. As a group, discussed the patient's presentation and identified clinical and care priorities.

7. Identified and shared one thing they learned from clinical rounds that day.

8. Reviewed their own and the group's performance, including feedback and suggestions for improvement in future group clinical rounds (steps 6 through 8 take ten minutes).

MUVE Setup

Setup for this learning activity requires careful and detailed preparation. The following elements must be planned and executed:

1. *Scheduling:* Scheduling this learning activity is done most effectively online. The activity leader can use a class web discussion thread to identify dates, times, and clinical focus for clinical rounds activity. Depending on class size and numbers of students participating, multiple clinical rounds sessions can be offered. Ideally, six students participate per group. Students can sign up for the clinical rounds session in an online discussion thread. For classes that meet in person, students can sign up on hard-copy paper or whiteboards.

Instructional Note: Students often ask to go to more than one clinical rounds learning activity on the same topic. This does not work very well as they have preexposure to the issues that will be raised in discussion.

2. *Location:* When students sign up for a clinical rounds session, the topic to be covered should be listed along with the date, time, and location for meeting. This learning activity requires four separate locations within a small area that is easy to navigate. First, students will convene for clinical rounds at a location that is easy to find. When using Second Life's® Second Health Hospital for the learning activity, the Polyclinic landing area is a good place to meet, as this area is right outside the hospital. The second location used for the assignment will be a nonpublic area in close proximity to the patient's location in the clinical environment. This could be outside the door to the patient's room or in the clinical area away from the patient where the group can discuss the patient without being overheard. The third location will be a clinical environment where the patient is located (clinic, emergency department, wellness center). In the last location, a few short minutes of postconference discussion takes place. Ideally, this is in close proximity to the patient's location but still in a place where discussion can be relatively private. It takes a bit of time for students to move their avatars from one place to the next, so these four locations should be as near to each other as possible. Early in the semester, I use the clinic sites just inside the hospital for clinical rounds because they are in close proximity to the Polyclinic landing area. This makes it easier for students to get to the learning activity location easily. As the semester progresses and students have developed their avatar walking skills, I utilize areas of the hospital that require covering more distance.

3. *Preparation of the Patient:* The instructor should make an avatar to serve as the patient for the learning activity. The avatar's gender, appearance, and so on can be modified to match the clinical presentation planned. Novice instructors may find it easiest for a teaching assistant or other instructional helper to act in

the role of patient. In this case, the activity leader should coach the assistant on what type of disease manifestation will be presented and what key issues he or she would like showcased in the patient's presentation. The patient avatar should be placed in the clinical location chosen for the learning activity and the assistant given the login information needed to log on, access the patient avatar, and proceed to the location where they will be interviewed by students on clinical rounds. They should wait there, sitting on a stretcher or sitting in a clinic interview area. They should do so a few minutes prior to the start of the learning activity to be in place and ready at the beginning of the activity. The activity leader can check in with them a few minutes prior to the beginning of the activity to ensure they are ready. This method relies on a clear written mini case study for the assistant to follow. An example of such a clinical presentation is as follows:

> Mrs. Jones is a newly married engineering student who has recently been diagnosed with systemic lupus erythematosus (SLE). She has come to the clinic for follow-up on abnormal renal function studies that her physician ordered as part of the diagnostic workup for her. Mrs. Jones knows very little about SLE and is focusing mostly on the fatigue that is preventing her from studying. Her grades are falling, and she has had to quit her job. At some point in the interview, she states, "I am just so stressed and exhausted that I can't think clearly and am having difficulty making decisions."
>
> Pertinent labs: positive SE factor, positive ANA, and slight elevation in BUN and creatinine.
>
> Elements to emphasize while acting out the patient role: fatigue and stress, inability to carry on life as usual (work, school, new marriage, etc.).

It is easier and in some ways preferable for the instructor to assume the patient role in addition to the activity leader role. It is not difficult to do this. The activity leader is most active in the first and last ten minutes of the clinical rounds activity, participating little in the middle ten minutes. The patient is active only in the middle ten minutes of the activity. There is very little overlap between the two, making it relatively easy to act as both activity leader and patient. It is easy to have two MUVE viewer screens open on one computer, one for the leader avatar and one for the patient avatar. The instructor moves back and forth between the two screens as the learning activity progresses. One significant advantage to doing the activity this way is that the instructor can control the patient's responses to students, making rich teachable moments possible.

Acting in multiple roles requires the activity leader to guide several avatars at the same time. It involves having two MUVE viewers open at one time, each taking up half the computer screen. On one screen, the instructor is logged in with the activity leader avatar. On the second screen, they are logged in with the patient avatar. (See "Tools to Use: How to Manage Two Avatars at One Time.") This method enables the instructor to control patient responses in a way that guides the conversation and creates learning opportunities. If a student asks the patient avatar an inappropriate question, for example, the instructor can have the patient respond in a way that is instructional ("How can you ask me that? That is too personal!"). This can create a learning moment that comes from issues that spontaneously arise. Some of the richest learning comes from these experiences! Once the instructor becomes comfortable with managing two avatars, he or she may decide to add a third. This avatar could be a consulting health professional such as a social worker or physical therapist who enters into the clinical rounds discussion. This can be an excellent way of illustrating the perspective of multiple care providers on the same patient.

4. *Creation of an evaluation rubric:* Once the clinical focus for clinical rounds has been selected, the activity leader identifies specific content that students are expected to apply in the clinical rounds activity. This is added to the performance outcome evaluation rubric for each participant. For each pathology studied, this can include the most important facts that a health professional needs to know about the pathology. It may also include pertinent lab values, suggested treatments, and drug therapy associated with the disease. The instructor should add professional role and interpersonal and group dynamics objectives that are expected to be applied during clinical rounds. The evaluation rubric can include a place for the performance of each student to be addressed, so grading from the activity transcript is easy once the activity is done. (See an example for a clinical rounds activity-grading rubric that focuses on SLE in Appendix 12 and a template-grading rubric for the clinical rounds activity in Appendix 13.)

Activity Procedures

1. The instructor will select a disease focus and write a brief case study description for the teaching assistant. Include the most important salient facts about the disease (no more than ten).

2. Identify a MUVE region location that is appropriate for the exercise (clinic, intensive care unit, emergency department, wellness center). Four total activity locations for the activity (described below) will be identified within the area chosen.

3. Prepare the patient avatar, changing appearance, gender, ethnicity, and physical appearance to match the clinical presentation (take into consideration demographic risk factors of age, race, and gender).

Instructional Note: As the instructor develops expertise with constructing avatars, he or she may begin to adapt the body of the avatar to match the clinical presentation.

4. The instructor will post the dates, times, MUVE region and location, and clinical focus for each clinical rounds session. The instructor should cap the sign-up at six (or five and one student activity leader).

5. The instructor next decides who will act in the role of patient. If an assistant is planned for the role, provide a clinical scenario and the login information for the patient avatar.

6. At the time scheduled for clinical rounds, the activity leader meets participating students at the meeting location. Because of the short duration of this exercise, students are encouraged to arrive inworld ahead of the scheduled time, so they are ready to begin on time. As the group is gathering, the activity leader assigns one of the participating students the responsibility of reminding the leader to copy the learning activity transcript when the activity is completed and before completing the learning activity. (In Second Life®, for example, the chat box is cleared as soon as all participants leave, so remembering to copy the transcript is crucial.)

7. Clinical rounds begin with the activity leader welcoming the participants and leading the group to an area outside the location where the patient is waiting. The leader asks the group what they remember about essential elements of the disease. The leader keeps track of the student responses, checking critical elements listed on the clinical rounds evaluation content rubric. After the students have finished giving their input, the leader adds any information from the rubric that the group has missed. This part of clinical rounds should take about ten minutes. A sample transcript of this first third of the clinical rounds activity can be found in Appendix 13.

8. After this introductory portion of clinical rounds is completed, the leader says, "OK, let's go talk with our patient." Students should be reminded that the patient interview will only be ten minutes long and that it does not entail obtaining a complete history, vital signs, and physical assessment. The group interacts with the patient with a goal of exploring the patient's experience and understanding of his or her disease, as well as some information about how having the disease has changed the patient's life. The leader should not speak during this period unless the group obviously needs guidance or if an error is

made that needs to be addressed immediately. At the end of ten minutes, the leader thanks the patient and leads the group back outside the clinical area to a private area where they can discuss the patient's condition. (For a sample of the second ten minutes of clinical rounds, see Appendix 15.)

9. Leaving the patient, the group reconvenes outside the patient's location in a nonpublic area where they can have a private conversation about the patient and his or her condition. The activity leader begins this part of clinical rounds with a question that focuses on some aspect of the patient's presentation. This question can vary a lot, depending on what the leader would like to focus on for the discussion part of clinical rounds. If the group, for example, had a good review of the pathology and focused on it well, the leader may choose to focus on a psychosocial aspect of the illness or patient teaching. Care planning should be the focus of this third aspect of clinical rounds. (See a sample of this last third of clinical rounds in Appendix 16.)

10. A few minutes before the end of clinical rounds, the leader should draw this portion of clinical rounds to a close and lead the group out of the clinical area into a place for a "postconference." For the last few minutes in this final location the leader asks questions such as "How did clinical rounds go today? What is one take-home piece for you?" This is a good time to affirm the "group brain," to restate that clinical rounds is a safe place to make mistakes (particularly if mistakes were made), and to affirm group learning. When students have completed their contributions, the activity leader thanks the group for their participation and closes clinical rounds.

11. The activity leader copies the clinical rounds transcript into a Word document. This should be distributed to the participating students and the instructor for subsequent evaluations using the clinical rounds grading rubric. The transcript can be posted for review by the whole class after deidentifying the learning activity participants. To deidentify students in the discussion use the "find and replace" function to replace student names with "Student 1," "Student 2," and so on.

Instructional Note: The activity leader should identify a student whose job it is to remind the leader to copy the discussion transcript from the chat box at the end of the group activity. Once the last person leaves the Second Life® area, the chat box is cleared and the discussion cannot be retrieved.

Evaluation

The clinical rounds grading rubric is used to evaluate the participation of each student as well as group performance. Summative evaluation statistics can be used both for evaluation of each student and for evaluation of MUVE clinical rounds activities in the course and across semesters (see Appendix 17).

For graduate-level courses and advanced role students, the assignment may be constructed so that students take turns being the patient and clinical rounds leader. In this case, evaluation criteria may be constructed to include the patient's ability to present a representative case study of a particular pathology and the leader's ability to effectively lead participants through the three stages of clinical rounds and the activity postconference. When these elements are included, role performance as activity leader and patient should be included in the clinical rounds performance outcomes. This option is a great way to develop clinical rounds leadership and case studies capabilities. It also frees the instructor to focus on evaluation and feedback.

Instructional Note: The success of this learning exercise is dependent on the activity leader's ability to focus on a small number of salient features of a disease for presentation in clinical rounds. For example, in the clinical presentation listed above, the activity leader could focus on the symptom of fatigue (very common in SLE) and the way that symptom contributes to the stress level of the patient. Clinical rounds could also focus on the role of stress and fatigue in SLE patients. Depending on the "patient," issues such as pregnancy (which can exacerbate both SLE flares and renal dysfunction) could also be included. Risk factors and issues related to lifestyle should always be included.

A sample description of the clinical rounds activity for use with the course syllabus may be found in the Appendix 18.

Final Comments: Most students love this learning activity. In the graduate pathology class I teach with clinical rounds as an extra-credit option, students often say, "This is where it all comes together." There is often a clear sense of team identity and "the group brain." Students often comment that because of the support of their group, they are not afraid to make mistakes and that, although very challenging, this learning activity is fun and energizing.

Tools to Use: How to Manage Two Avatars at One Time

1. In Second Life®, to operate a second avatar, first create a second avatar. The basic Second Life® account allows you to make multiple avatars. Every avatar created has a separate name. It is a good idea to label each avatar with a generic label such as Patient, Physician, Respiratory Therapist, and so on. This way the instructor can change the gender, age, and

appearance of each created avatar easily. (For names, the school name could be combined with the role name: for example, SONDHPatient.)

2. Log into Second Life®. On the drop-down menu on the upper left top of the screen, click on "ME," then "Preferences" and "Advanced Settings." On that screen, there will be an option to "Allow multiple viewers." Click on this and save the settings.

3. Minimize your current Second Life® screen. Adjust it to about half of your computer screen.

4. Keeping this screen open, click on your Second Life® icon or start up as if you are opening Second Life®. Log on with the "avatar" logon. Once logged on, similarly adjust the size of the screen to be about half the size of your computer screen.

5. Using more than two avatars at once is a little more complicated, and takes practice! What works best is keeping two screens "in play" at once, with the others reduced to a small size where you can enlarge them when needed.

Additional Resources

In the appendix section, there are a number of resources for this learning activity, including a description of the assignment that can be used for the course syllabus or for introductory material (Appendix 17) and sample learning activities for clinical rounds on asthma (Appendix 19), osteoporosis (Appendix 20), hyponatremia (Appendix 21), pituitary disease (Appendix 22), peripheral vascular disease (Appendix 23), and pneumonia (Appendix 24). Also included is template that can be used for planning a pathology-focused clinical rounds of your own (Appendix 25).

Reader's Roadmap: Where Are We?

Chapter 11 presented a complex small group learning activity. In Chapter 12, a second one is described in detail that enables participants to quantify and analyze their collaborative skills within a team.

CHAPTER 12

Sample Learning Activity 10 (Complex Small Group MUVE Learning Activity)

Building Small Group Consensus Skills

This chapter illustrates a complex MUVE small group learning activity. This illustration demonstrates how a MUVE learning activity can both support effective learning and achieve learning outcomes that are quite difficult to achieve using traditional methodologies.

This chapter is for you if:

1. You are interested in a specific sample of a complex MUVE learning activity.

2. You are interested in small group MUVE learning activities that focus on consensus building.

3. You are interested in MUVE learning activities that address pedagogical objectives more effectively than traditional teaching methods.

Sample Learning Activity 10: Developing Small Group Consensus Skills

Introduction and Purpose

This is a MUVE small group learning activity that combines small group MUVE activities, solo student MUVE activity, and both small and large group classroom activities to introduce, illustrate, and evaluate group individual and group consensus skills. This activity also illustrates use of a MUVE learning activity transcript in skill performance improvement. The purpose of this MUVE learning activity is to develop team collaborative skills in an activity that focuses on consensus-building skills.

INTRODUCTION TO COLLABORATION AND CONSENSUS

Collaboration is one of the most important skills professionals need to be effective in an interdisciplinary, globally connected world. Person-to-person, team, and broad organizational collaborative skills are crucial. Futurists who predict a postdisciplinary world where distinctions between disciplines become less distinct identify the importance of these skills as fundamental competencies for professional and interdisciplinary practice. Nowhere is this more true than among interdisciplinary health care professionals.

How are collaboration skills usually taught? If you are reading this book, chances are you are in a profession that requires collaboration. How did you learn it? Most of us learned collaboration by watching others collaborate and by trial and error in our own practice. Given how important this set of skills is for future success, we can and should do better. A MUVE learning activity gave me a chance to approach this important skill set in a new way.

Collaboration is a complex process that encompasses a wide range of skills. Collaborative skills are important for individual professionals but also as team skill set. Students learning collaboration need to understand its functional and structural importance in organizations, the nature of interdisciplinary practice, and the communication and interpersonal skills and attitudes necessary for successful collaboration. Students need to able to describe successful collaborations and also the consequences of unsuccessful ones. They must be able to assess and improve their own collaborative skills as well as those of the professional teams in which they work.

Ideally, in courses with a fieldwork or practicum component, students have assignments in which they are required to engage in a collaboration and afterward to reflect on it both theoretically and critically, including an assessment of their own strengths and weaknesses in the collaborative effort. Regrettably, such experiences are rare, and learning effectiveness in such practica varies greatly from student to student. Most such experiences lack objective measures for both learning and student performance. The theoretical component of collaboration is also often missing.

HOW CAN COLLABORATION BE TAUGHT?

Ideally, students would first learn collaboration theory and its application. They would learn about its importance, consequences of poor collaboration, and some specific examples of skills that are required for collaboration, such as consensus building. Then students would have a chance to work on the skills they have learned about. Students would be able to demonstrate skills associated with collaboration, have a chance to evaluate their skills, and plan for performance improvement in subsequent learning activities. Peers and instructor would offer specific feedback. A theoretical model would be used to help the student both understand the collaboration experience and use it in the evaluation process.

Using a MUVE to build collaboration skills can be done in just this way. What follows is an example of how a MUVE learning activity helped me teach collaboration, something that I had never been able to do to my satisfaction using traditional teaching methods. For this learning activity, I selected one of the specific skills necessary for effective collaboration: consensus building.

Target Population

This activity is appropriate for undergraduate- or graduate-level students. The activity works best in groups of five to seven students. It can be focused on discipline-specific collaborative groups such as nursing or medical students, social workers, or any discipline that requires work in teams. It is particularly effective with interdisciplinary teams working to improve interdisciplinary collaboration and team effectiveness.

Performance Outcomes

By the end of the learning activity, participants will be able to:

1. Describe three stages of consensus building.

2. Identify stages of consensus building in a series of small group discussions.

3. Identify the consensus stage in which they and each of their colleagues most participated. This is measured by the number of discussion entries.

4. Identify the consensus stage in which they and each of their colleagues least participated. This is measured by the stage in which the student contributed the fewest discussion entries. This indicates an area for development.

5. Identify "gems," defined as comments made by a group member that were particularly useful in helping the group come to consensus.

Through repetition of the activity:

6. Demonstrate performance improvement for an individual's weakest consensus stage, documented by evidence from a series of Second Life® learning activity transcripts.

7. Evaluate team performance in the consensus assignment, identifying specific areas for team improvement and demonstrating team skill improvement in subsequent consensus assignments.

MUVE Setup

This assignment progresses over two to three in-person meetings, interspersed with two or three Second Life® discussion group meetings (one before each class) and two written assignments. There is no specific MUVE setup required beyond assisting small groups in identification of an appropriate Second Life® meeting place. Health care administration students may want to meet in a business conference room, a health care team in a hospital conference room, and so on.

Activity Procedures

1. Students are divided into groups of six or seven students.

2. Consensus Discussion Group 1 (this takes place inworld): The small groups are given a topic to discuss as a MUVE activity. The discussion group goal is to develop a consensus response to a specific assigned question. One class was asked to discuss the ethical issues confronting people running small businesses and to identify the one that they thought was most important. There is no group discussion leader for this assignment. At the end of the discussion, one person in the group forwards the transcript of the discussion to each member of the group and the instructor.

3. Class 1 (in face-to-face class): In this class, the instructor presents a three-part model of consensus to the class. This model has three main stages. In the first stage, called the divergent thinking phase, the team's goal is to brainstorm and identify as many ideas as possible. For example, if the group assignment was to come to consensus on the most challenging ethical principle for people in business, the group would brainstorm possible examples of ethical principles that could be considered the most challenging. The goal in this stage is gathering diverse ideas, the more the better. In the second stage, the group identifies common themes among the ideas presented in first stage. In this stage, the focus begins to narrow toward consensus. In the final stage, characterized by convergent thinking, the group consolidates the various views discussed into a final single ethical principle.

4. After being presented this didactic material, the students discuss the theoretical framework to ensure they understood the differences between the stages.

5. The instructor then introduces written assignment 1. The class has an opportunity to ask any questions they have before planning their first MUVE meeting for the assignment.

6. Written assignment 1: Transcript analysis of Discussion Group 1. For this assignment, students are asked to begin their analysis of the Discussion Group 1 transcript by color coding the transcript. Each student in the discussion group is assigned a color. Using the color coding system, each participant codes the transcript with the colors for each group member. The students are then asked to analyze the transcript to answer the following questions:

STAGE 1 ANALYSIS

a. At what times did the group begin and complete stage 1?

b. How many minutes were spent in the stage 1?

c. What percentage of the thirty minutes was spent in stage 1?

d. Which student spoke the most in stage 1? Who spoke the least?

e. Were there any gems in stage 1 and, if so, who contributed them?

STAGE 2 ANALYSIS

a. At what times did the group begin and complete stage 2?

b. How many minutes were spent in the stage 2?

c. What percentage of the thirty minutes was spent in stage 2?

d. Which student spoke the most in stage 2? Who spoke the least?

e. Were there any gems in stage 2 and, if so, who contributed them?

STAGE 3 ANALYSIS

a. At what times did the group begin and complete stage 3?

b. How many minutes total did stage 3 take?

c. What percentage of the thirty minutes was spent in stage 3?

d. Which student spoke the most in stage 3? Who spoke the least?

e. Were there any gems in stage 3 and, if so, who contributed them?

Evaluation

Using the table below, count the number of times each member of the group contributed to each stage. Summarize in the comments column for each student the stage in which the student participated the most (presumed area of greatest strength) and the stage in which each student participated the least (presumed area in need of developing). Add a notation about any stage in which the student contributed a "gem."

Consensus Evaluation Chart

Student	Stage 1 Began at: Ended at:	Stage 2 Began at: Ended at:	Stage 3 Began at: Ended at:	
Student 1				Most entries: Fewest entries: Gems?
Student 2				Most entries: Fewest entries: Gems?
Student 3				Most entries: Fewest entries: Gems?
Student 4				Most entries: Fewest entries: Gems?
Student 5				Most entries: Fewest entries: Gems?
Student 6				Most entries: Fewest entries: Gems?

Instructional Note: Depending on the clinical rounds leader's preference, the data in this chart can be quantitative or not. It is very effective for students to calculate participation on a percentage of the total contributions that takes place in each phase. For example, if there are fifty entries for stage 1 and a student contributed twenty-five of them, he or she would have contributed 50 percent of the entries for that phase (can you say "air hog"?). It is most useful to use a combined quantitative and qualitative approach. The student who contributes the most gems may not speak very often. Similarly, a student who only speaks once but takes half the available time to do so would not be logged for too much participation if frequency only is analyzed.

Sample Completed Consensus Evaluation Chart

Student	Phase 1 Began at: 11:30 Ended at: 11:45 Total: 15 minutes	Phase 2 Began at: 11:45 Ended at: 11:50 Total: 5 minutes	Phase 3 Began at: 11:50 Ended at: 12:00 Total: 10 minutes	Phase Analysis: 50 percent of the time was spent in stage 1, very little time in stage 2
Student 1	11 entries	5 entries	2 entries	Most entries: 1 Fewest entries: 3 Gems?
Student 2	3 entries	4 entries	4 entries	Most entries: 2/3 Fewest entries: 1 Gems?
Student 3	2 entries	4 entries	6 entries	Most entries: 3 Least entries: 2 Gems?
Student 4	1 entry	1 entry	1 entry	Most entries: Fewest entries: Gems? 3
Student 5	5 entries	1 entry	4 entries	Most entries: 5 Fewest entries: 1 Gems?
Student 6	1 entry	4 entries	5 entries	Most entries: 5 Fewest entries: 1 Gems? 1

7. Class 2: This discussion can take place face-to-face or inworld. In this session, the groups divide into their discussion groups and compare their findings and conclusions. The following will be addressed: Was there agreement about the starting and ending times of each stage?

Was there general agreement about the individual performance of both group members and the team? Each group member will identify what he or she would like to do differently in the future. For example, student 1 spoke a lot in stage 1, but that meant that the discussion time allotted for collecting many divergent ideas consisted of mostly only her ideas. This may have effectively kept others from contributing their own. As a goal for the next discussion group, she might choose to speak less and/or invite and encourage the ideas of others. The group as a whole spent a lot of time in stage 1 and much less in the other two stages. The group could choose to even out the time in between the stages by identifying a timekeeper.

8. Consensus Discussion 2 (this takes place inworld): A second discussion topic is assigned for which the group is asked to come to consensus. The groups meet again inworld, complete the thirty-minute discussion, and distribute the transcript to each other and the instructor.

9. Written Assignment 2: The group will repeat the first written assignment. Added to the assignment is an evaluation of follow-up on the performance improvement goals they identified as individuals and as a group as a result of their Discussion Group 1 analysis.

10. Class 2 (face-to-face class): Each group presents their data to the whole group, summarizing what they learned and what progress toward goals they were able to achieve. Areas of improvement in the individual and collective performance of the group will be summarized, and progress toward meeting their goals will be discussed.

11. (Optional) Particularly in classes that do a lot of small group work, in MUVE or face-to-face, it is interesting to do a follow-up MUVE discussion group with a subsequent analysis to see if consensus behavior has continued to improve, leveled off, or deteriorated as the semester has progressed.

Evaluation

In this assignment, students participate in a 360-degree evaluation of individual and group consensus performance, based on objective data that provide an objective and theory-based foundation for feedback. Comparing data from their observations, students learn to compare data and evaluation conclusions. Both individuals and the group as a whole can plan performance improvement goals and follow up with further data collection and analysis to track progress toward goals.

Portfolio Evaluation

If portfolio evaluation is a part of the course, the learning activity transcripts and data summary charts, as well as narrative description of progress toward goals, can be included in the portfolio.

Reader's Roadmap: Where Are We?

This chapter completes Part II, which has offered specific examples of the types of MUVE learning activities introduced in Part I. The next chapter begins Part III, the "how-to" portion of the book. Chapter 13 begins by describing the first steps for designing a first MUVE learning activity, assessing personal, class, and organizational readiness for MUVE learning.

PART III

Planning, Designing, and Executing a MUVE Learning Activity

Part III focuses on specific how-to's for building MUVE learning into your teaching.

Chapters 13 and 14 address instructor, student, and organization readiness for MUVE learning. They review risk assessment and include a checklist for MUVE implementation.

Chapter 15 presents an orientation to Second Life® and provides specific guidelines for student and instructor orientation to MUVE learning.

Chapters 16 and 17 review design and implementation procedures for preparation of a MUVE learning activity.

Chapter 18 reviews special issues such as computer access.

Chapter 19 reviews common problems and pitfalls for MUVE learning as well as a discussion of preventive strategies and solutions.

Chapter 20 describes the development of an emotional intelligence course based on MUVE learning activities

CHAPTER 13

Instructor Readiness for MUVE Instruction

Taking the leap into MUVE learning can be both exciting and daunting. An instructor's first MUVE learning activity has the greatest chance of success if it is based on a careful evaluation of personal, student, and organizational readiness. The purpose of this chapter is to assist the prospective MUVE instructor in the identification of instructor and class characteristics that are necessary for MUVE learning activities to be successful. Risk assessment and optimum timing are discussed.

This chapter is for you if:

1. You have read Chapters 1 to 12 and are ready to begin laying the groundwork for designing your first MUVE learning activity.

2. You are interested in assessing indicators for course and instructor MUVE learning readiness.

Instructor, Student, and Organization Readiness for MUVE Learning

A few important features make planning for MUVE learning unique. If MUVE learning is new to your organization, assessing the right time to explore this innovation is crucial. If timed well, the first MUVE learning activity can be a success for your organization to celebrate rather than something that triggers the corporate immune system. Factors that support the best chances for success should be identified and strategically optimized. Risk factors for an unsuccessful learning activity must also be explored and considered carefully in the planning process.

The Best Time to Introduce MUVE Learning

The success of a first MUVE learning activity is largely dependent on a few essential issues that must be addressed. Successful MUVE learning depends on the following seven keys to success: the right teacher, the right course content, the right students, the right time, the right tech support, the right time for organizational innovation, and the right orientation. A discussion of the first two keys will be reviewed in this chapter. Keys 3 through 7 are reviewed in Chapter 14. In Chapter 15, orientation, the final key for success, will be discussed further.

Key 1: Are You the Right Teacher for a MUVE Learning Activity?

Even if you are fascinated by MUVE learning and eager to incorporate it into your teaching, it may not be right for you at this time. The following keys to success will help you understand what it takes to be ready for a successful first MUVE learning activity.

Dexterity with MUVE Skills

If you are planning your first MUVE learning activity in Second Life®, your own Second Life® skills need to be at a level that will enable you to design and execute a learning activity and also serve as the Second Life® resource expert for your students. You will need to guide your students through a Second Life® orientation, an orientation to MUVE learning, and an orientation specific to the learning activity you have planned. You will need to have the skills to assist students with a wide range of problems and issues that can come up at any stage of the learning activity. If you are struggling with any aspect of computers, Internet access, the Second Life® platform, or any aspect of the learning activity design, it is likely that the activity will not go smoothly. If you are having difficulty, it is likely that your students will as well.

Experience with Second Life® is crucial. If you are not yet comfortable with basic Second Life® skills, you may not be able to guide your students adequately or problem solve when they have difficulties. This can undermine learning and cause frustration even before an activity begins. During one of my first clinical rounds activities in Second Life®, my avatar became stuck inside a clinic wall. I continued to lead the activity as a disembodied voice coming from the wall. Because of the expertise they had developed in Second Life® and with their characteristic humor, my students were able to continue with the activity, but I never heard the end of it! In a less flexible or more novice group, this could have created a disaster. With more experience in Second Life®, I could have easily dealt with the problem and lessened its disruptive impact on the learning activity.

Instructional Note: It is likely that students will be using a variety of computers and operating systems. Make sure that your skills include use of both PCs and Macs, as the command system in the two differs. If you are not sure you are ready for MUVE teaching, the following suggestions may be helpful.

Get a MUVE Mentor

If you can, work with another instructor who has used Second Life®. Ask to observe a learning activity they have planned, or ask them to meet with you to talk about their own MUVE teaching. Even if they are from a different discipline, stories about their successes and failures, as well as suggestions they may have to offer, can be invaluable. If possible, observe one of their learning activities inworld. This will increase your familiarity with Second Life® and give you an opportunity to see another instructor's MUVE teaching.

As well as mentors, people who are enthusiastic about your MUVE teaching are important to cheer you through the difficulty of a steep learning curve. One morning, I led a MUVE learning activity in Second Life®. It was one of my first clinical rounds activities, and there was still a lot that needed improving. I was discouraged. Later that day, our nursing faculty member was scheduled to attend a lecture by nursing education innovator Dr. Patricia Benner. As usual, her talk was exciting and inspiring. At one point in her lecture, Dr. Benner asked for an example of contextualized learning. We were all pretty tired after a full week. No one answered. Nervously, I raised my hand and briefly described the clinical rounds activity I had just finished. "Wonderful!" she exclaimed, "You were tobogganing across the topography of the learning experience!" I was not totally sure what that meant, but she was clearly thrilled at the example and felt that it perfectly illustrated contextualized learning. I still have that sentence posted on my office wall. It continues to inspire me. In effect, her statement said to me, "I SEE what you are doing." That inspiration from a mentor like Dr. Benner has helped me through many difficult MUVE challenges.

Mentors Outside Your Discipline

Some of the most valuable feedback I have received about my own MUVE teaching has been from other instructors outside my discipline. The University of Hawai'i Center for Teaching Excellence is a department within the university whose mission is to help instructors improve their teaching skills. They offered instructional feedback in a variety of ways for my early MUVE experiments and provided wonderful support, encouragement, and feedback on my earliest MUVE learning activities.

Time Inworld Is Well Spent!

There is nothing like experience to make you feel more skilled. Nothing can replace time inworld. Explore Second Life® regularly using the MUVE skills you have. Look for opportunities to develop new ones. Make avatars and modify their appearance often enough to be good at it. Explore regions in Second Life®, including regions you would not usually visit and ones that on first look do not look appropriate for a learning activity. If you have a learning activity in mind, walk through it using the location you have planned for the activity. Do experiments, mock learning activities, or ones illustrated in this book. Make sure you are comfortable with your own inworld skills (walking, running, flying, teleporting, exploring a new site, sitting). Create problems for yourself. Throw yourself off a cliff, over a waterfall, or into an ocean and then get yourself out of that situation. From these activities, you will gain both experience and insight into the kind of problems students might encounter and how to work through them. Use the Second Life® Skills Checklist discussed later in Chapter 15. Add to it, building your skills gradually over time.

Instructor Teaching Style

Some teaching styles fit with MUVE learning better than others. A MUVE learning activity has structure but also lots of opportunity for students to mold their learning experience. Student agency abounds in MUVE learning! Surprises happen and a learning activity can suddenly move in a new direction. Some of the best MUVE learning activities I have designed mutated during execution into something unexpected and amazing. This requires instructors to have a flexible and open teaching style with a high degree of ambiguity tolerance. Flexibility that can accommodate a teachable moment is absolutely crucial. Instructors who cannot easily accommodate deviation from planned performance outcomes may have difficulty with MUVE learning activities.

Talking Story: The Learning Activity That Deteriorated into Something Amazing

One semester, clinical rounds in Second Life® was a weekly course requirement for a graduate-level course I was teaching. I was working with a particularly motivated group of students. They had done a few weeks of rounds and loved it. Their skills had improved steadily, and they were feeling confident. The level of energy in the group was especially high. Clinical rounds began with the usual review of the patient's specific presenting illness, a myocardial infarction (heart attack). The group moved enthusiastically to the patient interview. At this point, the students began rapid-fire questioning of the patient. Each student jumped in, one after the other, overwhelming the patient with questions. The patient was being interrogated. The students were relentless. I was acting the part of the patient and chose to abandon my plan for the presentation of a myocardial infarction and instead turn clinical rounds into a learning experience of a different kind. A teachable moment was at hand! I drew attention to the students' inappropriate approach to this patient by having the patient freak out at this onslaught. The patient began to cry, said she was overwhelmed, and reported that she was now having chest pain. In the activity leader role, I ended the patient interview and led the students out of the clinical area for post conference. "What went wrong?" I asked.

What followed was an amazing discussion among the students about the way their behavior had exacerbated stress and anxiety for the patient. The patient not only had been upset by their actions and the disruption of the therapeutic relationship, but also had become physiologically unstable. I concluded the last few minutes of the postconference debriefing by saying, "Every contact with a patient is an opportunity for healing. What will you do differently next time?" The students, who had been embarrassed and ashamed of their behavior, talked about what they would do differently next time. They also spoke about having made a mistake that easily could have been made with a patient in First Life. They had made a bad mistake in a safe place where no one was hurt. It was a mistake they would not forget. In clinical rounds for the rest of the semester, patient interviews had kindness and compassion as a main ingredient. The students had become aware of the medicine they could be to patients even in a short interview.

The Instructor and Course Content: Novice or Expert?

Instructor familiarity with course content is a crucial element that needs to be assessed prior to a MUVE learning activity. What is your experience with the subject matter on which the learning activity will focus? Are you a novice, teaching the material for the first time? Are you an expert with content mastery and little need to consult outside sources? Particularly early in MUVE teaching, it is important to select content for MUVE learning activities that you know well. The first MUVE learning activity that you do will be challenging enough! Your first MUVE activities have the best chance for success if they are supported by your comfort and expertise with both the activity's subject material and the course you are teaching. For your first MUVE learning activity, teach what you know best.

You want the first MUVE learning activity to have the best chance for success. A number of factors related to the class itself will optimize chances for a great first MUVE activity. Look for a class that could benefit from a simple one-on-one MUVE learning activity. These are the easiest MUVE learning activities to design and manage. If this type of activity does not make sense for the course content, it might be better to consider a different course for your first MUVE learning activity.

Failure Tolerance and Consequences

Early innovations are not always successful. The learning curve can be steep and slippery. If you are an instructor who easily learns from mistakes, has a positive attitude toward improvement, and can incorporate negative feedback into an opportunity, even a failed learning activity will not be problematic. "Get out there and fail," one of my nurse managers once said to her management team. She knew that trying new things, innovation, and new approaches involve periodic failures. It is important to assess the potential consequences of learning activity failure for your students. It is also important to assess your attitude toward failure and that of your supervisor. Would a failed MUVE learning activity be seen as a positive opportunity for improvement or a mark against the instructor?

Key 2: The Best Course for a First MUVE Learning Activity

The best course for a first MUVE learning activity is one that could benefit from a simple MUVE learning activity. Look for a class that could benefit from a simple one-on-one learning activity. These are the easiest MUVE learning activities to design and manage. If the course you are considering for a MUVE learning activity is already packed, it is less likely that there will be adequate time and energy for a MUVE orientation. The orientation itself will take several hours, and MUVE learning will take additional time and energy for the students to assimilate. Time pressure could lead to an unsuccessful learning activity.

In addition, a course that is already very full is not a good one in which to implement a new type of learning activity. Instructors must remember that students doing their first MUVE learning activity are accountable for both the learning activity itself and the additional MUVE learning curve as well. This adds additional burdens of time and energy. Students who already are feeling pressure in a chock-full course will not have a lot of tolerance for the additional energy and work required.

The Course That Will Benefit from the Pedagogical Advantages of MUVE Learning

A MUVE learning activity should offer students something that traditional teaching methods do not. If a learning activity in Second Life® makes the material come alive for a student in a way that traditional modalities do not, there is a good chance that the activity will be successful. A MUVE learning activity may help students overcome challenges related to language limitations, immaturity, social inhibition, or shyness. Students who have obstacles to expressing personal views may have a greater chance for success in a MUVE learning activity. An ideal course for a MUVE learning activity is one that will most benefit from what MUVE learning has to offer.

Courses with Content Challenges

Not all course content is riveting to students. Content that is dry, boring, or particularly difficult may be ideal for a MUVE learning activity. The positive energy MUVE learning generates may turn a dry, tedious course into one that energizes students. A course that students dread may be transformed into a fun one with MUVE learning. In one mandatory research course, a student who was open and humorous about her dislike of the topic in general reflected one day, "I can't believe it, I actually like this class!" For her, MUVE learning had made all the difference.

Tech Density?

Technology overload can be a serious problem for students. In classes using new technology, students effectively have two layers of course objectives to master. They not only have the challenge of the course content material itself but also the challenge presented by the technology being used to present course content. It is better to do a MUVE learning activity in a course that is otherwise relatively low tech. In such a course, all the energy students have for learning new technology can be applied to the MUVE learning activity.

Reader's Roadmap: Where Are We?

This chapter has addressed instructor and class characteristics that indicate readiness for MUVE learning. In Chapter 14, student readiness, timing, and risk assessment for MUVE learning will be discussed.

CHAPTER 14

Assessment of Students and Other Factors Related to MUVE Teaching Success

This chapter continues the MUVE readiness assessment with a discussion of student, organization, and technology readiness. It concludes with a checklist for assessing readiness for teaching your first MUVE learning activity.

This chapter is for you if:

1. You have assessed yourself to be ready for MUVE learning and would like to continue laying the groundwork for designing your first MUVE learning activity.

2. You are interested in assessing indicators for MUVE readiness that include student readiness, organizational and computer readiness, and assessment of risk.

Key 3: The Best Students for a First MUVE Learning Activity

If the instructor is clearly the right instructor for teaching a first MUVE learning activity and the course is ideal as well, there are other keys to consider. Picking the right students for a MUVE learning activity contributes to a successful first MUVE learning activity. The following elements should be included in this assessment.

Student Technology Skills

Doing a MUVE learning activity is far easier with a group of students who have already demonstrated technological dexterity or previous success with learning a new technology. For example, a group of students who made You-Tube videos for a previous class assignment have demonstrated the ability to learn and apply new technology. It is a good idea to survey students to explore attitudes and experiences with new technology before asking them to take the leap into MUVE learning. Student difficulty with learning new technology can be a significant obstacle to a successful MUVE learning activity.

Key 4: The Best Time to Implement a MUVE Learning Activity

Timing is everything! A MUVE learning activity has the greatest chance of success if it is introduced on a firm course foundation. Introducing a MUVE learning activity very early in a course may not be as successful as introducing it later in the semester. If the class feels secure with the course and comfortable with the instructor and they feel good about how the course is progressing, they will be more likely to be open to and successful with a new type of learning. Mid-semester is a perfect time to say, "Let's mix it up and try something a little different." The energy and interest a MUVE learning activity generates is often welcome in the mid-semester slump! Late in the second half of a semester is not ideal for a MUVE learning activity. At that point in the semester, student fatigue and stress are often high, and students have less energy for and patience with a new learning challenge. Workload is also typically heavier during the end of the semester, and additional work is neither appreciated nor appropriate. Additional work at an already busy time in the semester can produce negative attitudes toward MUVE learning that can undermine its success. Ideally, introduction of a MUVE learning activity occurs when both the students and the instructors have sufficient time and energy to adapt to MUVE learning.

Key 5: Are Computer, Internet Access, and Tech Support Adequate?

A MUVE learning activity should only be planned if there is adequate technology support for both students and the instructor. This is one of the deal breakers for your decision to implement a MUVE learning activity. There will always be technology problems. If a system is not in place for dealing with them, the credibility of the work is at risk. Realistically, sometimes the instructor is the only tech support available. In that case, the instructor is acting in two roles, instructor and tech support. In this case, the instructor must have sufficient time and expertise to perform both roles. This is not ideal. It is vastly better to work closely in partnership with an information technology (IT) team member. To evaluate the adequacy of tech support for MUVE learning activities, several factors should be considered.

Assessment of Tech Support for Instructor and Students

Before implementing a MUVE learning activity, a number of questions must be addressed. Who is available for the instructor if problems arise related to access to Second Life® or downloading it onto school computers? Who is available to the instructor to identify school computers that can be used for MUVE learning activities if a student's computer cannot accommodate Second Life®? If the instructor is planning to serve as tech support, who is available if there are questions or problems the instructor cannot manage? Whom will students call if they have problems downloading Second Life® or evaluating their computer's capability to support the Second Life® program? If students have tech difficulty during a learning activity, who will support them with problem resolution?

Adequate IT Support

It is best practice for an instructor planning MUVE learning activities to find an IT partner who is excited about learning in Second Life®. Such a partner can help navigate technology difficulties that arise and may also be willing to assist students directly as well. This can be challenging. If the IT department is not willing or able to support such a partnership, the instructor will need to make an assessment about the advisability of going it alone. Particularly for a first MUVE learning activity, the role of instructor will be challenging enough without adding the second role of tech support.

An IT team member may be available who is knowledgeable and interested in supporting MUVE learning but may not have time do so. A candid conversation with the IT team leader is important to assess this. If tech team members are available to help but do not know much about MUVE learning, additional training time might be necessary for them. Again, there is nothing like a good partnership between an IT team and an instructor doing MUVE learning activities. With flexibility, good communication, and a shared passion for MUVE learning, a great deal can be accomplished.

Computer and Internet Access

Unless the course requires students to have Internet access and/or a computer of their own, MUVE learning activities cannot be mandatory unless all students have access to a school computer. One way to deal with this is to ensure that the Second Life® program is available on computers in the student lounge, computer center, or library. It is crucial to identify this before planning a MUVE learning activity. Old computers in the library or lounge areas may not have sufficient RAM to accommodate the Second Life® software. Most relatively new computers do, but old computers are still around, particularly in lounges and libraries. If students are going to use those alternative computers, the instructor must check to make sure Second Life® is downloaded onto them and that the computers will be available during the hours in which MUVE learning activities will take place. For example, are the library, computer lab, or student lounges open in the evening or on weekends, when MUVE learning activities are most often scheduled?

Computer Requirements

Most computers less than five years of age can easily accommodate the Second Life® viewer and software support requirements. Occasionally, gaming software on computers or other RAM-intensive programs interfere with system capabilities. Students should be directed to other computers or encouraged to prioritize their RAM. As of the printing of this book, 1 GB of RAM was the minimum required to run the Second Life® viewer, and 3 GB is recommended. Smartphones cannot be used for MUVE learning activities. Some tablets can accommodate Second Life®, depending on their RAM capabilities. Tablets should be checked for individual RAM capabilities.

Learning activities in Second Life® should only be done on a secure web connection. Students should never use a wireless Internet connection for MUVE learning. This is important because even a very brief interruption in wireless connection causes the user to be logged out of Second Life®. The student's avatar disappears and the student must reopen Second Life® and log back in. The student not only misses part of the learning activity but the activity itself is disrupted.

Occasionally, institutional firewalls make it impossible to download Second Life® onto computers owned by the institution. Instructors should attempt to download the Second Life® viewer before beginning to plan a Second Life® learning activity. The IT department can often resolve firewall issues.

Key 6: Is It the Right Time for Innovation within the Organization?

One of the characteristics of professional maturity is an understanding that innovation, even on a small scale, affects the whole organization. The yeast of a small innovative project can expand to produce positive energy, excitement, and affirmation of both the innovator and the project. It can spread to other people, projects, and departments. At the same time, change, even on a small scale, can be perceived as threatening, a disruption of the status quo. It can, even on a small scale, generate negative responses from other faculty who disparage or discourage the innovator. If MUVE learning is new for your organization, there are a few additional issues to consider.

Risk Assessment

Not every MUVE learning activity works perfectly the first time. As well as the instructor's assessment of his or her own ability to fail constructively, planning the first MUVE learning activity should also include an assessment of the broader organization's relationship with innovation and failure risk. An organization, such as my own, that values innovation and has a high tolerance for steep learning curves is a safe place to try new things. An organization that penalizes failure poses a difficult challenge for any innovation, including MUVE learning.

Talking Story: Risk Assessment and MUVE Implementation

Before attempting my first MUVE learning activity, I did an extensive risk assessment. None of the faculty in my department had ever done a MUVE learning activity. Most did not know what a MUVE was. The IT support staff assigned to our department was interested and supportive but focused on other priorities. They simply did not have the time to help. My assessment of organizational readiness for MUVE learning included two big risk factors: the absolute novelty of the innovation and IT support limitations. However, there were also two positive organizational factors. Several other departments at the university were successfully doing MUVE learning. The university IT department had already addressed and managed potential problems for them. I had mentors and a support cadre of MUVE teachers available to me. They were passionate about MUVE learning and not only provided practical help but always left me encouraged and excited about the work.

Another deciding factor for my risk assessment was that my own department had a history of support for innovation. The dean was both interested in innovation and actively supported it. She knew that the road to innovation was a bumpy one. I felt sure that if my first MUVE learning activity was a disaster, she would support making the next one better. Best of all, when I described what my students could do in a MUVE learning activity, she was always enthusiastic and affirming. My organizational risk assessment contained both positive and negative factors. I decided to proceed with the design and implementation of my first MUVE learning activity.

Readiness Checklist

One way to assess the keys to success discussed so far is to review the following MUVE Innovation Success Checklist. There is no minimum score that indicates that it is a good time to begin MUVE. The process of completing the checklist and reviewing it with an organizational supervisor or mentor can help identify both supporting factors and obstacles. This process will help instructors come to conclusions about overall readiness for MUVE learning activity implementation that will give it the best chance for success.

MUVE Innovation Success Checklist

Assessment Criterion	Your Assessment	Comments
1. Is this the right time for you as an instructor to begin your first MUVE learning activity?		
2. Are the students the right students for a successful first MUVE learning activity?		
3. Is this the right course for beginning MUVE learning?		
4. Is the timing right for implementing MUVE learning?		
5. Is there adequate tech support for instructor and students?		
6. Is this the right time for the organization to embrace MUVE learning?		
7. Is an adequate orientation possible for students new to MUVE learning?		

Key 7: Is the Right Orientation Possible?

The last question that must be addressed before moving forward with design and implementation of a MUVE learning activity is, "Can students be provided with an adequate orientation to MUVE learning?" If students are unfamiliar with MUVE learning, before they can be asked to participate in a MUVE activity, they first must "learn how to learn" in a MUVE. This is a crucial issue, another potential deal breaker for your first MUVE learning activity and one that involves many topics worthy of discussion (see Chapter 15).

Reader's Roadmap: Where Are We?

Part III began with a discussion of risk and readiness assessment, the first important phase of designing and implementing a MUVE learning activity. Chapter 15 continues with the issues raised in Key 7: orientation to MUVE learning.

CHAPTER 15

Orientation to Second Life®

Chapter 15 describes issues related to orientation to MUVE learning in general and, by way of an exemplar, to Second Life® orientation in particular. This chapter supports orientation to Second Life® but could be used as a guideline for an orientation to any other MUVE, as basic functions are similar and similar issues need to be addressed. This chapter will include a Student Second Life® Orientation Checklist, elements included in the Instructor Orientation Checklist, and discussion of special issues such as privacy and griefing.

This chapter is for you if:

1. You are interested in reviewing an existing instructor or student orientation in preparation for teaching a MUVE learning activity.

2. You are interested in developing your own instructor or student orientation materials in preparation for MUVE teaching.

3. You are planning to use a MUVE other than Second Life® and are interested in exploring key elements of orientation of students and instructors to MUVE learning.

Second Life® Orientation: In Class, on Paper, and in the Syllabus

This chapter will review important issues and elements for orientation to Second Life®. The issues discussed and skills outlined in this chapter can also be used to create an orientation to any MUVE. A MUVE learning activity can only be successful if students have an opportunity to complete an effective introduction and orientation to MUVE learning. They must be given the opportunity to develop the skills necessary to function in a MUVE prior to being assigned a learning activity. Ideally, the orientation is spiraled through the course, with key points repeated several times. Students need to be exposed to important concepts multiple times and through multiple media. For example, the importance of using a wired Internet connection (not a wireless connection) can be emphasized when the instructor introduces MUVE learning in class, later when a specific learning activity is introduced and in both the written activity description and the course syllabus. Although MUVE activities work best when scheduled for the middle of a semester, the instructor can begin talking about MUVE learning as soon as the course is under way, so the orientation begins slowly and the class gradually becomes familiar with, and excited about, MUVE learning.

The course syllabus must contain a description of MUVE learning activities planned for the semester. Performance requirements for each MUVE learning activity can be listed in the syllabus or in attached MUVE materials. The MUVE materials for the course ought to include a written MUVE learning orientation, a detailed introduction to and instructions for every MUVE learning activity that takes place in the course, and grading matrices for each learning activity. A sample introduction to Second Life® for students is included in Appendix 26.

Detailed outlines of student and instructor orientations to Second Life® are included in Appendixes 27 and 28. It should be emphasized that simply completing the instructor orientation checklist does not mean the instructor is ready to design and implement a MUVE learning activity. Other important issues, such as those described in Chapter 13, must be considered, as the role of a MUVE learning activity instructor goes beyond specific skills. Problem solving, managing change, working with tech support issues, and other elements are all necessary for successful design and implementation of a MUVE learning activity.

A comprehensive assessment of whether a sufficient orientation can be provided for students is an absolute deal breaker when it comes to making the decision to do a MUVE learning activity. If students cannot be adequately oriented to MUVE learning, they cannot be expected to be successful in MUVE learning activities planned for them. Ideally, discussion of MUVE learning begins early in the course, so students can gradually assimilate the knowledge, attitudes, and skills that they will need for MUVE learning activities later in the course. Particularly students who have obstacles to learning with new technology may require additional encouragement, redundant orientation, and face-to-face sessions with the instructor to be ready for MUVE learning.

Materials to Support Second Life® Orientation

Student Second Life® Skills Checklist

Students working in Second Life® must be able to download the Second Life® software, create a Second Life® account, make an avatar, and then, inworld, learn to walk, sit, teleport, use the chat room, and be able to copy a chat room discussion into a Microsoft Word document. Additional skills such as sending a postcard may be needed for specific learning activities. One orientation goal is that students not be overwhelmed with required MUVE skills. It is very important that the technology not interfere with learning. It is important to keep required MUVE skills at a basic level.

At the beginning of orientation, the instructor tells the students how much time is allocated for Second Life® orientation. For a basic orientation and mastery of the skills listed above, two to three hours are more than sufficient. The instructor should emphasize that skills beyond those required, such as avatar appearance or clothing, are not included in the time allotted for orientation. Students should be provided with a skills checklist specific to the MUVE platform being used. The first MUVE learning activity assigned can include completion of the checklist, including a student signature to indicate confirmation of skills mastered. If a portfolio evaluation system is used for the course, a copy can be added to the course portfolio.

Instructional Note: It is very important that students use their real first name and a fictional second name when they create their Second Life® account. If students do not use their real first name, it can become difficult to keep track of their activity in Second Life®. This rule must be introduced early and reinforced several times. It is a good idea to identify students with the same first name and ask them to use the name you suggest. Two students named John could be JohnS and JohnB. It is very difficult for an instructor to keep track of alternative names, so some time and attention to this issue will save an instructor time and energy later on. To preserve student privacy, a student's last name should never be used.

The Instructor Second Life® Skills Checklist

A comprehensive Second Life® basic skills checklist for instructors is included in Appendix 28 but should be considered only a reflection of baseline skill level, not a terminal goal. The instructor's orientation to Second Life® is a continuous learning process of expanding and improving in skills. This is an important part of being a MUVE instructor. A student will be required to do only a few basic skills, but an instructor must be master of not only basic skills but also more advanced ones. The instructor must also be an effective resource for problem solving and be able to provide assistance for students having difficulty. Additional skills that instructors must have relate to instructional design. Instructor orientation to Second Life® teaching includes both specific skills (how to rescue a lost student) and management of processes (how to troubleshoot lag). Among the required skills for being an instructor for MUVE learning activities are the following:

Moving around the MUVE

The instructor must be a master navigator. Developing the ability to move around the MUVE easily takes some time. When an instructor is orienting students to Second Life® or leading a learning activity, students look to them as an example. If the instructor avatar moves easily around the environment and negotiates obstacles, looking comfortable and proficient, students will model this performance. If the instructor is awkward, hesitant, or having difficulty moving the avatar, student learning will be distracted and their confidence undermined. Remember, this is outside many students' comfort zone. It is as if they have been taken to the moon to learn! The instructor's ability to project confidence and ease will reassure them and make learning easier. Also, again, the technology must not distract from the learning! Students overly absorbed in figuring out how to sit or watching the instructor struggle to make his or her own avatar sit will have less attention and energy for learning. The technology will have undermined learning.

Locomotion skills include walking, running, and flying around complex environments. The instructor must be able to climb stairs, go up elevators, and move around trees and other objects in the environment. While you are in the MUVE, envision the kinds of problems students might have. What if a student tries to fly and get stuck in midair? How will you help him or her? As you encounter problems, think about how you would help a student in the same situation. How would you help if a student gets stuck in a tree, wall, or some other object? What if a student falls down a waterfall or cliff, or falls into a body of water? These things do happen and can significantly disrupt a learning activity. The more dexterity an instructor has in negotiating such problems, the better a learning activity's chances for success.

The instructor should also be comfortable teleporting from one MUVE region to another and from place to place within regions. Many regions are large enough that visitors are offered means to move from one area of the region to another by teleporting. At the main landing area of the region, maps or other structures assist with teleporting to other areas of the island ("Click to teleport to the beach area," for example).

The instructor can also practice rescuing students who get lost. The best way to do this is to send the student an invitation to teleport to the instructor's location. See "Tools to Use" at the end of this chapter on how to do this. The instructor must be familiar with this procedure and practice it prior to the first orientation or learning activity using a second avatar in a split screen.

Communication: The Chat Box and Transcript Skills

The course instructor must be dexterous with every form of communication available in the MUVE being used. The recommended form for Second Life® learning activities is the chat function. The instructor must develop the habit of copying the chat box contents into a Word file at the end of every student activity, so that a record of each activity can be kept. If confidentiality is a concern, the Word "Find and Replace" function can be used to replace each student with a numerical identifier or other designation. For some learning activities, students benefit from being able to review discussions from other small groups. If such discussions are intended for distribution to the entire class, such redesignation of names in the transcript is recommended.

Instructional Note: It is a good idea for an instructor to copy the transcript at the end of every MUVE learning activity in which the instructor is present, even if a student has been assigned to do so. Loss of a transcript because someone forgot to copy it can be a disaster. Ensuring there is a backup copy of the transcript is good insurance. This also can reinforce the instructor habit of copying transcripts every time, as instructor loss of a transcript (for example, an exam transcript) can be equally disastrous. Once the last participant has left a chat and logged off, the dialogue from the chat box is cleared of all but a few entries. For some learning activities, it would be necessary for students to repeat the learning activity if a transcript were to be lost.

Second Life® Instant Messaging

When using Second Life®, the instant message (IM) function is important for the infrequent situations in which it is necessary or desirable to communicate with a student during a learning activity privately and directly. This could be the case in the event of inappropriate behavior, for example. Also, if a student is lost, sending him or her an IM to check in may be the only way to communicate with that person if he or she is more than thirty (inworld) feet from the group or lost in another region. Messages using the IM function do not appear in the chat box transcript and are not logged, so there is no documentation of their contents. For this reason, use of the chat as exclusively as possible is preferred.

At the start of orientation and in their first learning activity, students need to be reminded to use the chat function to communicate, not the IM function. A mix of the two for a learning activity does not work, as not all students can see IM entries. Also, the IM messaging is not included in the activity transcript.

Instant messaging can result in confusion and an incomplete activity transcript. It must be reinforced repeatedly that only the chat box is used for the learning activity.

Controlling the Second Life® Environment

If utilizing Second Life®, the instructor should be aware of a few issues related to specific Second Life® environments. It is important that the instructor be able to deal with issues related to regional lighting, lag, privacy issues, and environmental factors that can interfere with learning. Regional lighting and lag will be addressed in the following section. Privacy issues and environmental factors that can interfere with learning will be explored in Chapter 19.

Regional Lighting: Changing the Time of Day to Be Conducive to Learning

Second Life® is on a day to night cycle lasting four hours, with three hours of daylight and one of night. This means that it is possible for a user to log into Second Life® during daylight (bright light), early morning or evening (muted light), or even at night (dark with only moon and artificial light). Night lighting is not appropriate for most learning activities, so it is important to know how to adjust a region's lighting to a time of day that best accommodates student learning.

Tools to Use: How to Adjust Regional Lighting

To change the time of day depicted, look at the upper left edge of the Second Life® viewer, where you will see a series of words for drop-down menus. Click on "World" and, at the bottom of the drop-down menu, select "Sun." The menu that appears offers a selection of times of day. The selection "noontime" offers the most light and is in most cases the best for a MUVE learning. However, for a learning activity whose goals include fostering interaction and intimacy, such as a getting to know your discussion group at the beginning of a semester, evening light or sunset may create an ambiance that will support this goal.

Instructional Note: If participants arrive in Second Life® at night, each must change the regional lighting on his or her own Second Life® viewer. This should be addressed in the orientation for students, as the instructor simply changing the lighting on his or her own viewer will not change the settings for individual students. If an instructor is present for a learning activity and notices it is night, it is good practice to guide the students present with the steps necessary to adjust the lighting conditions.

Managing Lag

The instructor must be prepared to manage lag. Lag is defined as a delay that sometimes occurs in some MUVE processes. Lag in a MUVE can manifest as visual images that take a long time to rez, or appear, particularly when an avatar teleports and arrives at a new location. The avatar itself may not appear immediately, taking longer than usual to rez. A particularly troublesome form of lag is the delay in the appearance of clothing as an avatar rezzes! This can be disturbing to the users, as what they see first is their unclothed avatar. At no time do these avatars appear naked to others in the environment. Instead, they appear as a semiformed cloud, only a shadow of the avatar form.

Lag can also appear as a delay in movements or actions for things in the MUVE, such as slower movement of a car or boat. A delay in communication is one of the most troublesome consequences of lag. This is usually experienced as a delay between the time words are typed into the chat box and when they appear to other participants. These words won't appear in the conversation on time, in an appropriate sequence. Rather, they pop into the conversation so late that they can seem inappropriate. A more detailed discussion on lag will take place in Chapter 19.

Creating an Avatar and Avatar Appearance Modification

A critical instructor skill for designing MUVE learning activities is the creation and use of avatars. Although students usually use only the premade avatars (unless they choose to modify their avatar's appearance on their own time), the instructor must be expert at the creation and adaptation of avatars for use in MUVE learning activities.

The Instructor Avatar

Instructors should begin by being thoughtful about the creation of their own avatar. Inworld, instructors must be professional role models. This applies to how they behave and treat others, but also in their appearance. Instructors can intentionally present an appearance similar to what they would wear in First World to class or on campus. An instructor can alternatively present an appearance that strategically supports the goals for MUVE learning. For example, I am a professor at the University of Hawai'i. The dress code in Hawai'i is quite casual, and organizational relationships, both in the workplace and in the academic setting, are more relaxed than is the case in other parts of the United States. Because I did not want the informality of a digital representation of myself to potentiate this cultural informality, I designed my avatar to be formal and businesslike in appearance. My avatar wears a black suit, a white shirt and tie, and, sometimes, a lab coat. My title, Professor Codier, floats over my head. These visual cues reinforce professional relationships, the role of instructor, and a degree of formality to offset my digital appearance.

Use of Multiple Avatars

Complex learning activities may require a group to interview a patient or have a discussion with a physician or social worker. To that end, a second avatar can be constructed. Naming of the avatars for use in learning activities was reviewed in Chapter 9. It is a good idea to ensure that the names are gender neutral (UHPatient, not UHPatient Mrs. Jones). This way, from week to week, the avatar's ethnicity, age, and gender can be changed as needed. It is better for students in rounds to meet each time with a patient whose name is "Patient" rather than "Mrs. Jones" who presents with a different disease each week! It is also a good idea to begin an avatar password file so you do not forget the names of additional avatars' logons and passwords.

Modifying an Avatar's Age, Gender, and Ethnicity

Creating an avatar (a patient, for example) for use in a learning activity, whose appearance contextualizes and enriches the learning activity, is a crucial element of designing avatars for a MUVE learning activity. Intentional illustration of risk factors or high-risk groups for a particular disease can support case presentations of specific diseases. Selection of gender and ethnicity can be accomplished by changing the avatar's body. In Second Life®, this is accomplished by clicking on the "people" icon at the top of the column of icons on the left-hand side of the Second Life® viewer. Clicking on this icon will present a selection of avatar bodies to select from. Most of the avatars are twenty to forty years of age in appearance. To create the appearance of an old or very young avatar, additional changes need to be made by modifying the avatar's body or by having the avatar "wear" an older or younger "skin."

Changing the Avatar's Body Shape

Modification of the avatar body is a great way to make the avatar better illustrate the disease he or she is presenting to the class. In Second Life®, alterations in body shape can be made by right clicking on the avatar and selecting "Modify shape." Using the drop-down screens that appear, parts of the body can be thickened (to make swollen ankles for a patient with congestive heart failure [CHF], for example). To make a patient appear cushingoid, you can make his or her trunk and abdomen thick, shorten and thicken the neck, and make legs and arms long and thin. An avatar can be adapted to look emaciated, obese, and so on. This takes some trial, error, and creativity! Once the changes are made, they can be saved. By saving changes to an avatar's body in their inventory (for example, clothes can be saved), the instructor can create a whole library of avatar appearances (a CHF patient, a patient with systemic lupus). To make an avatar look older, shrink the size of the shoulders, lengthen the neck, make the head taller and more narrow, and so forth.

Remember the goal is that the appearance of the avatar should offer visual cues that support the learning activity narrative! This takes some practice.

Changing an Avatar's Age

Changing an avatar's age is one of the important changes to make in Second Life® avatars, which nearly all appear to be in their twenties. Some "skins" (these are like masks that can be added on to an avatar body) are available that can make the avatar look older or younger. Narrowing the shoulders, thinning the hair, and elongating the neck can all make the avatar look older. For children, a "child skin" is the easiest way to portray an avatar child.

Changing an Avatar's Clothing

If the clothing an avatar is wearing does not work well for the purposes of a learning activity, clothing can be added to the avatar's inventory (the suitcase icon along the left-hand side of the Second Life® viewer). Many locations in Second Life® offer free clothing, including the orientation island where avatars are born. Newly acquired clothing can be worn immediately or saved for future use in the inventory under the heading for clothing. Some alterations in the body itself (rashes, amputations, bleeding wounds) are also possible, as are the addition of assistive devices (wheelchairs). These items can also be saved in the inventory for future use.

Reporting Griefing

Sadly, there are Second Life® residents who find being disruptive to others a source of entertainment. Second Life® is a public place that is not policed. Inappropriate behavior, called "griefing," has consequences for the perpetrator if individual users take responsibility for reporting poor behavior. Instructors must be familiar with how to report griefing. Reporting griefing is not included in the basic Second Life® skills list, and in general, the instructor should take responsibility for creating the griefing report. I have found that a report from an instructor from a learning activity that was disrupted is taken very seriously, not only by the Second Life® managers but also by the owners of the region where the griefing episode took place. Students should be taught about griefing, and they should be asked to make a note of the time and location of any griefing as well as the name of any avatar that disrupts a learning activity or bothers them in any way. This can be taken directly from the learning activity transcript, which is a good record of the griefing event. Managing griefing will be discussed in Chapter 19.

Skills for Maintaining Privacy in Public Space

The instructor must develop skills to support MUVE learning privacy in what must be considered a public space. Methods for maintaining privacy in a public space require constant adaptation. Such skills include identifying MUVE regions that both provide appropriate context for the learning activity (a hospital, a classroom, a clinic) and at the same time enforce both student patient information privacy. This important issue will be discussed in depth in Chapter 19.

Setting Limits

It is important that instructors reinforce with students that they are responsible for only basic MUVE skills and that they are not required to modify their appearance, change clothes, and so on. Students may choose to do so, but this should be considered "on their own time." The MUVE worlds are fun, diverting, and interesting, and it is easy to get a little carried away. I confess I spent the better part of a weekend early on in my MUVE teaching trying to make my avatar's hair move as the avatar walked! It is important to set limits on the fascinating parts of the MUVE world that, while interesting and diverting, are not necessary for learning activities.

Tools to Use: How to Send an Invitation to Teleport to Your Location (Student Rescue)

Occasionally, a student gets lost, teleports incorrectly, or otherwise becomes separated from the learning activity group. To accomplish a rescue the instructor can:

1. Using the search window in the Second Life® viewer, search for the student's inworld name.

2. When the name appears, the window will include an option that states, "Offer teleport."

3. Click on this option.

4. In the student's viewer, an invitation to teleport to the instructor's location will appear.

5. When the student clicks on the teleport invitation, he or she will immediately be teleported back to the instructor's location.

Reader's Roadmap: Where Are We?

This chapter used orientation to Second Life® as an exemplar for issues related to any MUVE orientation. The next chapters, Chapters 16 and 17, will focus on the design, planning, and implementation of a MUVE learning activity.

CHAPTER 16

Designing a MUVE Learning Activity, Part I

Readiness for MUVE Learning

Building on the readiness assessments covered in Chapters 13 and 14, the next two chapters review the design and implementation of a MUVE learning activity.

This chapter focuses on specifics of learning activity design and implementation. The next chapter discusses integration of a MUVE learning activity into a course. Progressive levels for integrating MUVE learning into a class are outlined.

This chapter is for you if:

1. You are planning your first MUVE learning activity and would like to explore both how to design the activity and the issues related to activity design.

2. You want to improve a MUVE already in use.

3. You want to develop systematic skills for designing a MUVE learning activity.

Planning the Design of a MUVE Learning Activity

One way to design a MUVE learning activity is to answer a series of questions related to the structure and design of the learning activity itself.

Question 1: Should the Learning Activity Be Simple or Complex?

Considering the student and instructor characteristics for this course, where should the MUVE learning activity fall on the continuum of simple to complex? MUVE learning activities can be very simple or very complex. They can also be highly unstructured or highly structured. It is advisable to begin with a simple, relatively unstructured MUVE learning activity. With a relatively simple activity, the instructor can practice basic MUVE instructional skills (student orientation to MUVE learning, implementing MUVE learning within a course, problem solving technology issues) and at the same time practice working out any unexpected problems related to teaching as a novice instructor.

TWO ENDS OF THE SIMPLE-TO-COMPLEX CONTINUUM

The importance of assessing instructor and student characteristics to determine the appropriate complexity for MUVE learning activities is well illustrated by MUVE learning activities used with two very different groups. The first was a group of health care technicians. They had a primarily passive learning approach and did not have much experience with reflective thinking or critical analysis. They were not accustomed to thinking with the group brain. Many expressed resistance to online learning in general and described themselves as low tech.

With this group, I had planned optional MUVE discussion groups for the later half of the course, but I was unsure of both the group's baseline computer skills and their readiness for new ones. I was aware of considerable group resistance to online learning. For this situation, early in the course, I selected a mandatory MUVE learning activity that was simple and unstructured, with very few points allotted to its grade. I made it mandatory so I could assess the students' skill level in a relatively low-risk assignment. The learning activity I chose was a one-on-one "getting to know you" MUVE session. Pairs of students met for thirty minutes in a MUVE and interviewed each other with a series of questions designed to help the students to learn about each other. Beyond answering the questions, there were no structured requirements for the assignment.

To my surprise, the group made a game of overcoming their technology phobia. Students who were nervous paired with students who weren't. This playfulness reduced overall resistance to MUVE learning. The students helped each other, and after that first assignment, most of the class chose to continue with the optional MUVE learning activities that were offered later in the course. For this group, the selection of a low-risk, simple, unstructured assignment that had a very small role in the overall class made it possible for students to be successful with later, more complex and important MUVE learning activities. It also engaged students who were resistant to this type of learning because it was low risk, fun, social, and easily accessible.

On the other end of the simple-to-complex continuum was a small class of graduate-level nurse clinical specialists in the second semester of a two-semester online class whose focus was application of pathophysiology to clinical practice. All but one student had been in the first semester class in which

I had successfully used many MUVE learning activities. Student performance outcomes had been excellent. By this time, I had taught hundreds of MUVE learning activities and considered myself an expert. I wanted to take the next step in my MUVE teaching by offering highly complex, very structured, and mandatory MUVE learning in a course taught almost entirely in a MUVE. The student group was small, MUVE experienced, highly motivated, and tech savvy.

I chose to design the course to take place almost entirely in a MUVE. The graduate students in the class participated in MUVE discussion groups, one-on-one client interviews, group clinical rounds in the MUVE hospital, and all course exams there as well. In these activities, students were able to apply pathophysiology content, practice professional roles, and apply both interpersonal and teamwork skills in a simulated environment. The activities had very specific performance objectives and specific criteria for each objective. All of the course credit was dependent on MUVE learning activities, so the stakes were high. As it turned out, the course was highly successful. At the end of the course, students reported that although the course had been very hard, the learning was outstanding. The choice of complex learning activities was appropriate to the students, the instructor, and the content focus for the course.

These two examples represent the continuum of options for planning mandatory MUVE learning activities, from a course using a simple unstructured one-to-one learning activity to one that involved many learners in complex multilevel learning.

Question 2: Which Specific Course Objectives Will Be Addressed in the MUVE Learning Activity?

The specific course objectives that will be addressed by the MUVE learning activity are selected to maximize the impact of the activity. The instructor makes use of pedagogical synchrony to match the learning activity with the objective it best addresses. Since the advantages of MUVE learning include contextualizing learning, developing colleague and team skills, and using the group brain, the course objectives selected for the MUVE learning activity should emphasize these. For example, even if the learning activity is content focused, the learning activity should still include interpersonal and team function objectives.

Question 3: Which MUVE Learning Activities Are Most Appropriate for Meeting Course Objectives?

Selection of the type of MUVE learning activity (solo, one-on-one, or small group) that is best suited to the course learning objectives includes several issues. First, the level of MUVE experience for teachers and students must be considered. If either are fairly limited, a solo or one-on-one learning activity is most appropriate. If team skills are to be addressed, obviously a small group activity is indicated.

As well as course content and methodology, the interpersonal, team, and professional skills related to the course objective must be considered. An example was a MUVE learning activity for novice clinical nurse specialist (CNS) and nurse practitioner students who had not done much interviewing at an advanced level. The MUVE learning activity had two objectives. The first was that the students practice interviewing, and the second was that they would learn how to do a focused interview for a patient with a particular disease. This is a good example of a dense learning activity. The students applied course content (what should be included in a focused assessment for a patient with CHF?), skills development (interviewing), and also role development (how is interviewing different in student, clinical nurse, nurse practitioner, and CNS roles?).

Instructional Note: MUVE learning performance outcomes should be specific and measurable. One way to ensure this is to link every objective for a MUVE learning activity with an item on the grading matrix. Make sure it is easy to read the activity transcript and check off the performance outcomes on the grading matrix you have designed.

One of the strengths of MUVE learning is that in the simulation of virtual space, there is a vast opportunity for students to apply not only content but also interpersonal and team skills, continuous learning, and emotional intelligence skills. The learning activities can be very dense, incorporating many dimensions of learning at once. Make sure that the MUVE learning activity performance outcomes reflect this!

Question 4: Where in the MUVE Will the Learning Activity Take Place?

LOCATION, LOCATION, LOCATION!

For some MUVE learning activities, location does not exert a major influence on the learning activity. For example, one-on-one "getting to know you" activities can take place pretty much anywhere. Students often enjoy picking their own locations for these activities. Indeed, locating a good place to talk develops MUVE skills like walking, searching, and teleporting. Even in these cases, it is a good idea for the instructor to provide examples of places students might try out. This is a particularly important for students who are new to the MUVE you are using.

For most MUVE assignments, however, the MUVE environment will greatly contribute to learning effectiveness. For example, a small group that will be meeting together all semester for an ethics discussion may have a first getting to know you session. If this takes place around a campfire or at the beach, the intimate environment may help support students be more open with each other. Other environments simulate the context in which learning will be applied in the future. If the assignment involves a nurse practitioner interviewing a client, the learning is contextualized when the activity takes place in a hospital or clinic. Situating the learning activity within an appropriate context enhances learning and subsequent translation of learning into clinical practice. This contextualization of learning is one of the greatest strengths of MUVE learning. Care should be taken to situate MUVE learning activities appropriately.

The instructor will need to spend time exploring the MUVE find locations that are appropriate for the goals of the learning activity planned. Hospitals, clinics, offices, and other environments would be suitable for health care learning activities. Other MUVE learning activities are strictly dependent on a specific environment for which the learning activity was specifically designed, for example, the content-rich environments discussed previously.

BUILDING YOUR OWN LOCATIONS

Often instructors beginning to use a MUVE make the assumption that they will need to build their own learning environments. Building learning environments is awesome work that requires a high level of MUVE technical mastery. It also is expensive in time, money, and other resources. Designing and building an environment is a full-time job. Remember, lots of places in MUVEs have already been constructed and are available to use. Particularly in the beginning of MUVE teaching, it is important to focus designing and implementing MUVE learning activities that can take place in regions that already exist. If a new region must be constructed for a particular learning focus, partnership with a construction specialist is recommended.

PRIVACY

Unless a region is privately owned and closed to public users, there is no guarantee of privacy in MUVEs. Nevertheless, there are several ways to make a learning activity private enough to support effective learning.

For all MUVE learning activities, consider locations where there is not a lot of public activity. For example, meditation islands and gardens foster group intimacy and sharing. They are wonderful places to conduct discussions and team simulations. These locations do not usually have many people in them, so there is relative privacy. In public MUVEs, highly populated, popular regions, there are more people simply wandering around. Learning activities in these locations have a higher chance of people listening in out of curiosity. At best, privacy in these regions is more difficult to maintain. At worst, individuals may disturb the group and interfere with the learning process. Even the interruption of individuals who are genuinely interested in being included in the activity takes a few minutes to deal with. Popular sites are also more apt to have lag because of the number of people on site. Lag, privacy, and griefing will be discussed in more depth in Chapter 19.

Question 5: What Are the Specific Steps for the Learning Activity?

After identifying goals for the learning activity, the number of participants, and the location, the instructor should map out specific procedural steps for the learning activity, from the earliest step to the last piece of documentation. This constitutes a to-do list for every MUVE learning activity. Although instructors may devise their own personal checklist, a basic one follows:

CHECKLIST FOR PLANNING A MUVE LEARNING ACTIVITY

1. Assess instructor strengths/weaknesses for teaching this learning activity.

2. Assess the target student population strengths/weaknesses for engaging in this learning activity.

3. Evaluate how much technology support may be needed for the learning activity as well as technology support availability.

4. Where will this learning activity be on the continuum of simple to complex?

5. Where will this learning activity be on the optional to mandatory continuum?

6. What are the learning objectives for the learning activity? (Include specific content, communication, interpersonal, and group skills.) What specific performance outcomes are involved?

7. Devise an evaluation matrix for the learning activity based on the learning objectives and specific performance outcomes.

8. On the basis of steps 1 to 7, write a brief description of the learning activity for distribution to students. Make sure that the steps for involvement in the learning activity are very clear and that each participant

is clear on what is expected of him or her. The grading matrix should be attached and responsibilities for self-evaluation, peer evaluation, and/or group evaluation included.

9. Write the syllabus description of MUVE learning for the course, including a brief description of each MUVE learning activity. If the activity is mandatory, computer requirements should be included and alternate computer access described.

10. Identify, if appropriate, the MUVE region that will be used for the learning activity. (Note: it is essential for the instructor to visit the region before the learning activity takes place. Changes in the region that occur without the instructor's knowledge could negatively affect the learning activity.)

11. Prepare and distribute MUVE orientation materials. Repeated orientation in class is preferable. The more students hear about the MUVE, the better (see Chapter 15).

12. Review students' avatar names to ensure that there are no duplicate avatar names in the class. If students have not used their actual first name, they should be asked to rename their avatar. It is not acceptable to expect that the learning activity participants know that "Baby Bunny" is actually Susie under an assumed name. Mismatched names can cause great confusion in a learning activity and should not be permitted.

13. If the assignment involves student sign ups (discussion groups, volunteer leaders), this should take place at least a week prior to the due date. This will give time to fix problems that arise in the sign-up process.

14. For all group leaders, voluntary or assigned, provide specific direction as to what is expected of them.

15. Make sure it is clear to the participants who is responsible for sending the transcript of the learning activity to the instructor (a lost transcript is a catastrophe—it is not retrievable in Second Life®, for example, once the group has logged off).

16. Set up a system for logging participants and logging grades and extra credit from evaluation matrix forms.

17. Devise a system for combining the learning activity evaluation matrices into a summative evaluation for the activity and for course MUVE activities.

18. When the learning activity has been completed, review transcripts, complete grading, provide feedback, post grades, add extra credit points, and complete other documentation as needed.

19. Complete your own review of the student performance overall and share with the class. If not all class members participated, invite MUVE learning activity participants to share what the activity was like in class.

20. Complete a self-evaluation of your MUVE teaching. What did you learn from doing this learning activity? What would you do differently next time? Include this evaluation in the file with the learning activity materials so your own suggestions can be incorporated into the activity the next time you do it. Include: What is the logical next step to continue developing your MUVE teaching skills?

Just as instructors use a set of procedural steps for building and implementing a MUVE, students can also be given procedural steps for doing a MUVE learning activity. This can help students new to this kind of learning organize their first MUVE assignment. The following is an example of steps for student participation in a MUVE learning activity.

PREPARING FOR A MUVE LEARNING ACTIVITY

The week before the MUVE learning activity is planned, all students should:

1. Download the MUVE software, if needed

2. Open an account if this is required for the MUVE platform you are using.

3. Make an avatar, using as the first name the school abbreviation (UMCDavid) and using your first name as the avatar second name. Note: students must *not* use their full names, but it is essential that they use their first name. This ensures they can be identified by peers and the instructor. If more than one person in class has the same name, the instructor should discuss this with students involved. Sometimes a nickname or abbreviated name is preferred by the student and would work as a good substitute name. Avatar appearance should be professional, including human form and dress similar to what would be appropriate in the classroom or in the clinical setting.

4. Send the avatar name to the instructor.

5. Practice the following (and ask for help if you need it):

   Teleporting from one area to another

   Walking and moving around objects

   Communicating using the chat function

   If transcript capability is available on the MUVE platform, copying the chat transcript and pasting it into a Word document

6. Review what to do if the learning activity is disturbed. (Remember, begin with "This is a university learning activity, would you please allow us some privacy.")

7. Review the learning activity and be clear ahead of time what is required. Get in touch with the instructor if there are any questions.

8. Teleport to the MUVE location where the learning activity will take place. It is a good idea to go there well ahead of time and log off of the MUVE while at the meeting area for the learning activity. When logging back on the next time, the avatar will be located where it was when logged off, ready for the learning activity to begin.

9. Log on to the MUVE ten minutes ahead of time, ensuring readiness to begin the learning activity on time.

Reader's Roadmap: Where Are We?

In this chapter, the first stage of implementing a MUVE learning activity was described. In Chapter 17, a strategy for integrating a MUVE learning activity into a course will be explored.

CHAPTER 17

Designing a MUVE Learning Activity, Part II

Implementing MUVE Learning

This chapter reviews the strategic considerations for integrating MUVE learning activities into a course. Included are such topics as making an activity mandatory or optional and ways to progressively course MUVE learning activities from optional to mandatory gradually as a way to deal with student resistance or negative perceptions of new learning technology.

This chapter is for you if:

1. You are designing a MUVE learning activity and are interested in a guide for strategic integration of the activity into a course.

2. You are interested in a systematic and staged way to develop your own MUVE teaching skills.

Integration of MUVE Learning Activity into a Course

Once an instructor has concluded that it is the right time to teach a MUVE learning activity, that the class content is a good match for MUVE learning, that the students have a good chance to be successful in MUVE learning, and that there is both adequate technological support for the activity and sufficient time for orientation, it is time to start planning. Planning for successful MUVE learning begins with strategic decisions about integration of MUVE learning into a course. How will the MUVE learning activity fit into the course? Will it be a mandatory activity or an optional one? These questions must be considered as the instructor makes strategic decisions about integrating MUVE learning into a course.

Optional or Mandatory?

It is recommended that an instructor begin MUVE teaching with an optional, very informal MUVE learning activity with a small number of interested, motivated, and tech-savvy students. Over time, in later courses, instructor can increase the number students in MUVE activities he or she is planning. This can happen gradually as instructor skill and comfort level increase. Eventually, the instructor will be ready for a whole class to be involved in mandatory MUVE learning. Gradually increasing the number of students as the instructor shifts MUVE learning from optional to mandatory enables the instructor to gradually increase the number of student problems and degree of resistance he or she manages. This enables the instructor's own MUVE skills to improve gradually.

Levels for Gradually Integrating MUVE into a Class or an Instructor's MUVE Teaching

Level 1: Try an optional learning activity "on the fly"

Level 2: Take one small step: The optional assignment

Level 3: A MUVE learning activity as an extra-credit option

Level 4: A MUVE learning activity as an alternative to an existing assignment

Level 5: The "no thank you" MUVE assignment

Level 6: The mandatory MUVE assignment

The following is a progression of levels an instructor can use to develop MUVE teaching skills from the relative ease of an optional MUVE assignment to a more demanding mandatory assignment. It can also be used as a road map for gradual integration of MUVE learning into a course or across time with a particular group of students progressively developing MUVE learning skills.

LEVEL 1: TRY AN OPTIONAL LEARNING ACTIVITY "ON THE FLY"

Sometimes taking a leap and trying something on the fly can be a great way to begin. The circumstances need to be right and the risk low. My own experience has shown that this can be a great experience.

Talking Story: Trying It on the Fly. One semester, I was concerned about a small group of highly motivated overachievers in my class. I felt that they were bored and increasingly disinterested as the rest of the class plodded along covering some pretty difficult course material. The small group was beginning to check out. It was time for me to take action or risk losing both their interest and their contributions to the class. I had been considering offering an optional extra-credit MUVE learning activity later in the course but decided it might be fun to challenge the small bored group with it right away instead. At that point in the course, the class was doing small group discussions. I offered anyone in the class the option of doing the discussions in MUVE instead of face-to-face. I offered MUVE orientation sessions and the group began. Most of the bored group participated. They loved it and asked to continue the mandatory weekly discussion groups in MUVE. They actively recruited classmates to join them. Their enthusiasm was infectious. They sold MUVE learning to their peers by sharing their experiences with the rest of the class, who got curious (and a little jealous). When it was time to offer the optional MUVE learning activity later in the course, not only was the class already interested and eager to join in, but I had a core of students who were happy to lead the discussion groups and mentor those who needed assistance.

LEVEL 2: TAKE ONE SMALL STEP: THE OPTIONAL ASSIGNMENT

The first formal step into a MUVE learning activity should be one that does not involve the whole class and is voluntary. The advantages are as follows:

1. There will be a small number of students involved since an optional assignment will not appeal to the entire class. This makes a first MUVE learning activity easier for the novice MUVE instructor to manage.

2. Students who volunteer are typically motivated and energized. If not sold on MUVE learning, they are at least open to it and have a positive overall attitude. This means that the instructor can focus energy on activity design and implementation. Less time will be spent on having to sell the idea to students who may be resistant, uninterested, or need a lot of support with new technology.

3. A small MUVE learning activity with a few students gives both instructor and students a chance to deal with unexpected problems more easily than if they are happening to the whole class at once.

4. With a small, less formal MUVE learning activity that involves only a few students, the stakes are lower. There is less pressure on instructor and students. If the activity is not a total success, the negative impact is minimized.

5. Feedback from a small number of participants is easier to solicit and manage than getting it from a lot of students all at once. How many times does the instructor need to hear "There was not enough orientation?" before they know they need to revise their activity plan?

LEVEL 3: A MUVE LEARNING ACTIVITY
AS AN EXTRA-CREDIT OPTION

A MUVE learning activity offered for extra credit has an excellent chance of success. Students are often motivated to do whatever it takes to get extra credit. This should not, however, be the first MUVE learning activity that an instructor attempts. Students who want extra credit the most are often students who are not performing well in the class. Their grades are low and they need extra credit. This is not the ideal student for a first MUVE learning activity. They are motivated, but not necessarily for reasons that may make them successful in MUVE learning. In addition, even students with good grades often want extra credit, and an instructor may find there are more students wanting to participate than the instructor has resources or time for.

Nevertheless, there are good reasons to do a MUVE learning activity for extra course credit. Students who want extra credit are indeed highly motivated. Given the chance to improve their grade (which often gives them a sense of control and hope—student agency is a powerful thing), these students often are motivated to complete the MUVE orientation and do as much MUVE learning as they can. The extra motivation helps them sail through the orientation and gives them extra impetus to solve any particular problems that come up during orientation or early MUVE learning. Some of the best-performing MUVE learners I have worked with were those who badly needed extra course credit. Many of these students also reported that they learned better in MUVE activities. A MUVE learning activity for extra credit not only may give struggling students extra credit but also may provide them with a way to learn that may be more effective for them.

I discovered this when it became apparent that students who did not need extra credit were attending extra-credit learning activities. The same thing was happening with lower performing students who had maxed out on the amount of extra credit they could receive but continued to sign up for optional MUVE learning activities. When I asked them about this, both groups responded with comments like, "This really helps me learn" and "This is where it comes together for me." Although extra-credit MUVE assignments do tend to attract a lot of students, it is unlikely that everyone in the class will participate, so once again, a smaller number of students will likely be involved in the activity.

LEVEL 4: A MUVE LEARNING ACTIVITY AS AN ALTERNATIVE
TO AN EXISTING ASSIGNMENT

This is a useful next step for some of the same reasons extra-credit assignments are a good early step into MUVE learning. A MUVE learning activity alternative to an existing assignment will not typically appeal to the whole class, which means that it will involve a smaller number of students and therefore be more manageable. Making a MUVE learning activity available also enables students to select a learning modality that works best for them.

Students usually report that, once they have completed MUVE orientation, they spend less time completing MUVE assignments compared with other learning activities. The efficiency of time and resources appeals to many students. Students report that they can be more flexible and economical with their time and resources with MUVE learning. This makes sense considering what it really takes to do a small group discussion in person. Face-to-face groups involve time spent dividing the class into groups, having them physically move to the area where the group will meet, sitting down and getting organized, and then gradually getting down to work. Students who do MUVE learning activities perceive that it is a more effective use of their time. At the agreed-upon time, students log into the MUVE and the activity begins nearly immediately. Because students know the session is recorded in a transcript, they get down to work quickly. They tend to accomplish group tasks more effectively. Because they know their participation will be evaluated, participation is more even qualitatively and quantitatively across the group. Based on my observations over years, MUVE activities take roughly 50 percent less time than equivalent face-to-face activities to achieve the same goals.

Offering a MUVE activity as an alternative to a regular assignment also helps manage student resistance. If students come into class with resistance on the basis of preexisting negative attitudes ("I heard you do this Second Life® thing in this class, which I can't do because . . ."), it is a good strategy to offer the MUVE learning activity as an alternative to an assignment that students usually don't like or find difficult. Students may overcome their own resistance to a MUVE learning activity if they view it as a preferable option.

Instructional Note: If a series of optional MUVE learning activities are offered throughout a course, it is preferable to let students opt in or out of them at any time. This option involves more logistical work for the instructor, but it can be worth the additional signup and tracking time. In one series of weekly discussion groups, as the weeks went by, more and more students chose to do the MUVE discussion group. Students in the MUVE groups recruited and mentored their friends. The energy and fun of the groups became contagious. This ended up being better for the students because more students got the experience of learning in virtual space, and learning outcomes were far superior. It was also beneficial to the instructor. Beginning with a relatively small group of MUVE learners and then gradually increasing the number of students over time enabled me to gradually increase my MUVE learning activity management skills.

At no point did the MUVE teaching seem overwhelming. This is a great way to keep the project manageable and gradually build MUVE teaching skills.

LEVEL 5: THE "NO THANK YOU" MUVE ASSIGNMENT

Remember when you were a child who didn't want to try a new food at dinner? Did your mom ever insist that you have a "no thank you" portion? This serving consisted of a tiny pile of whatever it was you didn't want to eat. You had to try it, but you didn't have to eat much. Sometimes, you hated it. Sometimes you found a new favorite food! The no thank you assignment is like that.

The no thank you assignment can be a good approach for a first MUVE assignment that will take place in a series over time, for example, weekly discussion groups. With this approach, the instructor tells the class they all have to orient to MUVE learning and do one MUVE discussion group, but after that they can choose a face-to-face discussion group if they prefer. There are some advantages of trying this assignment approach prior to MUVE learning activities later in the course. After doing the "no thank you assignment," the one small mandatory MUVE learning activity, some students who thought they would not like it find out they do. When students who have a great deal of resistance to a MUVE learning activity are told, "You only have to do it once . . . if you don't like it, you don't have to continue," their resistance usually decreases. After the assignment is completed, some of the resistant students find they did like it and continue with MUVE work. The others who prefer not to do MUVE work still had the experience of learning outside their comfort zone, which is in itself beneficial. The "no thank you" approach in a mandatory assignment, paradoxically, gives students a sense of control that supports their learner agency. Sometimes they find out they really like the new "food"!

LEVEL 6: THE MANDATORY MUVE ASSIGNMENT

A mandatory MUVE learning activity is not necessarily any better than an optional one, but sometimes for pedagogical reasons, it is desirable to have the entire class involved in the activity together. For learning activities that are very complex and are dependent on a known number of participants, a mandatory activity is often preferable. When a course is presented entirely in a MUVE or has objectives that can only be met in a MUVE learning activity, the mandatory option is necessary.

Reader's Roadmap: Where Are We?

Chapters 16 and 17 have reviewed the design, implementation, and strategic issues related to integrating MUVE learning into a course. In the next chapter, Chapter 18, several special circumstances for implementing MUVE learning are discussed, including using MUVE learning when students do not have their own personal computers and using MUVE learning to improve an existing course.

CHAPTER 18
Special Topics

The purpose of this chapter is to discuss three special topics for MUVE teaching: improving a MUVE already in use, using a MUVE learning activity to improve a traditional class, and MUVE learning for students without computers or with limited Internet access.

This chapter is for you if:

1. You are interested in improving a MUVE that you are currently using.

2. You are interested in using a MUVE learning activity to improve a traditional class.

3. You are interested in using a MUVE learning activity with a class with limited computer or Internet access.

Improving a MUVE Currently in Use

If you have already designed and implemented a MUVE learning activity and want to improve it, the following steps may be used to assess the activity and plan for its improvement:

1. Begin with what students said about the learning activity after they completed it. Include all written evaluations and anything students may have said informally. If you can, communicate with students from previous classes who did the same activity ("I will be doing the MUVE learning activity again. Do you have any suggestions for how to make it better?"). As consumers of MUVE learning, nothing is more important than student perceptions about what did and did not go well. If there is a formal student evaluation at the end of the course, review it for any mention of MUVE learning and include these data in your summary.

2. Evaluate in writing what you think did and did not go well. Include the resources required for planning and implementation, including

how much time and energy were required for you and the participants. Think about the activity from a big-picture perspective. Did it energize the course or deplete energy? Did it seem like a good fit with the course or did it break the flow of learning? Were there any surprises? In the end, was it worth the effort? Did it accomplish anything a traditional learning activity could not?

3. Evaluate the learning activity against the twenty steps for creating a MUVE learning activity outlined in Chapter 16. Were there steps missing or incomplete? This may indicate weak links in the chain of your activity, identifying areas you could improve.

4. Evaluate the learning activity objectives. Were they specific and clear? Were they multidimensional, including interpersonal or team process ones, or did they only reflect application of course content? Did completion of the objectives meet your intentions for the activity? Were unforeseen objectives achieved? Are there objectives you would like to add, expand, or clarify for future use?

5. Evaluate the technology aspect of the activity. Did use of this technology support learning or distract from it? Were there technology obstacles to learning? If so, were there recurring problems (Internet access, computer limitations)? Did students get needed technology support? If the instructor served as technology support, did it interfere with the instructor role?

6. How were learning outcomes evaluated? Was a grading rubric used? Did students do self-evaluation, peer evaluation, and, if appropriate, evaluation of group function? Was portfolio evaluation used? Were summative and formative evaluation data collected? Was there anything you would change in the future on the basis of the data gathered?

   Use an evaluation matrix to collect performance data. I like to review it with a peer, mentor, or supervisor as a foundation for making plans for upcoming MUVE learning activities. This is particularly important if there is organizational resistance to your utilization of this technology or if MUVE learning is new to the organization. This evaluation can also be added to your own professional portfolio as a way of tracking the effectiveness of your MUVE learning proficiency over time. This quantifies the effectiveness of MUVE learning and can demonstrate its value.

Summarize Your Evaluation: On the basis of this summary, what specific changes will you make for the next time the learning activity is offered?

Using a MUVE Learning Activity to Address a Learning Challenge in a Class Taught with Traditional Methodologies

A MUVE learning activity can also be used to address specific learning challenges for classes taught with traditional methodologies.

Online Learning and the Sense of Presence

The demand for learning that is financially and geographically accessible is increasing. Part of this demand comes from students who work but are interested in higher education. More students in the United States are seeking graduate-level education than ever before. These students are often employed, and many have family responsibilities. Most are interested in learning that is independent and self-directed. Online courses are a perfect solution for these individuals. Students around the globe who are seeking continuing education but have limited academic access similarly rely on Internet learning. Although the body of research on learning effectiveness and best practices for teaching online is still in its early stages, Internet-based learning is here to stay.

One serious drawback to online learning is that the sense of presence students experience face-to-face in a traditional class is often lost in the online venue. Many online classes do not require live interaction between students. Even discussion groups for these classes are often asynchronous. This is a problem because group learning, teamwork, and the creative synchrony that occurs when students interact are very difficult to experience online. A MUVE learning activity creates this sense of presence as students, in their avatar forms, meet in real time to work together. Group learning, social support, creativity, experiencing the group brain, and teamwork skills are all activated by MUVE activities. Students very often report that the sense of presence they experience in MUVE learning is a very positive influence on the course.

Talking Story: The Pathology Class

I was teaching a class that was essentially a hard-science, content-driven class. This class had little in the way of interpersonal work or content related to relationships, communication, teamwork, or group dynamics. I had added MUVE learning to the class essentially to break up the dryness of the material and enliven its application. The MUVE activities for the course consisted of small groups engaged in a variety of activities together ranging from discussion groups to group projects. The participants were from all over the globe. At the end of the class, I got an e-mail from one of the international students. She said, "So, when are we doing the group debrief and closure session?" Honestly, I thought she had sent the note to the wrong professor. Surely, she was referring to a clinical group or psych class, in which the bonding of the group throughout the course requires an intentional closure process at the end of the semester. When I wrote back to clarify, she simply said, "We have all gotten really close in our inworld meetings. The course study group became our support system." This was one of those moments when I was simply stunned at the secondary effects of what I thought was a straightforward content-driven MUVE learning activity.

Relationships and Learning

For many students, strong group relationships and a sense of team identity support learning effectiveness. The emotional and social engagement of one-on-one relationships supports learning. This is true particularly for students who externally process, engage emotionally in the learning process, and process their intelligence using their interpersonal and intrapersonal intelligences. For some course content, this interpersonal and group engagement is crucial for achieving the course's objectives. For example, a professionalism class that includes objectives related to self-care, teamwork, burnout prevention, or stress management will involve a lot of personal sharing. The quality of this sharing will be improved if individuals within the group get to know each other and feel comfortable sharing and thinking through issues together. For groups that form a sense of group identity, a learning activity can become a crucible within which the group's work is deeper and its impact more comprehensive. MUVE learning activities support this development of group and individual relationships. They also support the development and growth of group identity. Relationships in the group develop as participants do things together and learn about each other through shared experience.

Instructional Note: It is worth noting that the sense of presence activated by MUVE learning is largely a function of students' relationship with their avatar. As mentioned in the prologue, one of the differences between online gaming and MUVEs is that in a MUVE, the avatar is an extension of the users' presence. The answer to the question, "Are you your avatar?" seems to be yes!

Talking Story: Avatar Presence

My primary field of academic research is emotional intelligence (EI). I got into MUVE learning because I was looking for better ways to teach EI abilities (see Chapter 20). I was at an EI conference presenting my ideas for teaching EI in MUVE settings. As I stood up to give the presentation, one of the psychologists present, one of the senior members of the group, made a negative comment about the whole idea. He said it in a joking way, but it was clear that he did not think much of my plan. I laughed, and said, "Maybe I can change your mind," and began my presentation. I talked about an avatar as an extension of a person. "My students from an isolated geographic region have no one to talk to about their professional growth," I said. In a MUVE learning activity, a student becomes an active member of a dynamic community. I went on to describe the power of MUVE learning to help students change behavior, experiment, and try out new ways of being. The avatar is not a substitute for traditionally personal or face-to-face relationships. It is, rather, an extension of a person. The group caught on to the excitement of possibilities that MUVE learning offers. At the end of the presentation, the elder psychologist who had bad-mouthed this idea before my presentation stood up, beaming, and simply said, "I am sold!"

Integration of Emotions in Learning

There is increasing interest in the role of emotion in learning. The role of emotional experience in the learning process has become a subject of interest as the scope of learning effectiveness research incorporates emotional intelligence and other theories about intelligence into new pedagogical approaches. There are some who go so far as to say that learning itself is in its essence an emotional process. The experiential, interactive, interpersonal, and group possibilities that MUVE learning offers are fueled by positive emotional experiences, relationships, and group support. This is one of the most compelling reasons for MUVE learning and one of the most rewarding to witness. Of the hundreds of small group learning activities that I have evaluated or witnessed, very few conclude without a strong sense of group energy and identity. This mobilizing of this positive emotional energy is one of the outstanding characteristics of MUVE small group learning.

There are many examples of the integration of emotional abilities into MUVE learning activities. Some MUVE learning activities involve the development of emotional abilities as a secondary effect of a broader learning goal. For example, a MUVE interview activity in which a student interviews a client who is grieving may have a primary goal of using knowledge of the grief process to effectively communicate with a person who is grieving. The skill of empathetic communication may not be the primary goal of that activity, but it could be a secondary goal that is met as the primary goal is achieved. Other learning activities may target the development of emotional skills themselves. The following is such an example.

Sample Learning Activity 11: Rewriting History

Introduction and Purpose

In a class focused on developing emotional intelligence ability, students were asked to complete an assignment called Rewriting History. This assignment took place after the early portion of the course in which students had learned about emotional intelligence competencies and had begun to explore how to develop their own.

Target Population

This activity works as a one-on-one or small group activity. It is appropriate for any level of student. It is particularly effective when used in an interdisciplinary setting.

MUVE Setup

There are no particular setup requirements for this learning activity

Performance Outcomes

The evaluation matrix for this activity includes the application of one of the four primary emotional intelligence abilities to the activity. Depending on the level of the learner, self and peer review can be added to the performance outcomes.

Activity Procedures

1. Students are asked to write the story of an emotional interaction that occurred at any time in their lives in which the emotional outcomes of the interaction were unsatisfying.

2. For the second part of the assignment, students meet inworld to share the story with another student and to discuss in emotional intelligence terms what went wrong during that past interaction. In the MUVE session, students share ideas about how one emotional intelligence ability could be used to rewrite the story.

3. In the final portion of the assignment, students review the MUVE discussion transcript and then write a dialogue of the reimagined

event to illustrate how a different outcome could have been achieved. They use an emotional intelligence ability to "rewrite history."

Evaluation

This assignment can be evaluated several ways. The creativity of the "rewrite" may be the focus of the evaluation. If a more quantitative approach is required, the operational definition of emotional intelligence may be used and the four emotional intelligence abilities applied to the students' rewrites.

Instructional Note: The objectives of this MUVE learning activity primarily focus on applying knowledge of emotional intelligence competency to a specific situation, and also to continuing the development of peer relationships and peer coaching skills. Students may use painful experiences from their lives involving someone important to them or a minor, relatively trivial encounter. As students report their rewrites of history, they often describe this rewriting of history as a healing experience. Even imagining how the experience could have been different seems to have a positive impact.

One of the most valuable aspects of learning activities in MUVE is the ability to try new behavior in a safe place in which the cost of failure is low and the chances of harming anyone else are negligible. The opportunity to make rookie mistakes in a virtual simulation rather than with a live patient makes student clinical learning with patients safer. It may also make for a higher baseline competency level for entry-level practitioners beginning practice. The ability to trial new personal behaviors, experiment with a new conflict management style, or try out new emotional intelligence abilities similarly offers students a way to try out new behavior in a safe place, where the emotional and interpersonal cost of failure is low.

Using MUVE Learning Activities When Student Computer and/or Internet Access Is Limited

It seems counterintuitive to use MUVE learning in a classroom where the students could as easily be doing face-to-face learning activities. However, some of the benefits of MUVE learning (the ability to document small group activities, interview dialogue, disinhibition) are so useful that a class sitting together in a computer lab, doing a MUVE learning activity, may be an excellent idea. If students in a class do not have access to personal computers or the Internet, using computers in a school learning lab or computer science lab for MUVE learning activities is a good solution. This can be an alternative use of class time that can provide both a change of pace for the face-to-face class and the pedagogical advantages of MUVE learning.

Reader's Roadmap: Where Are We?

This chapter reviewed the use or MUVE learning in special circumstances, such as using MUVE learning to improve an existing course. In Chapter 19, problems and pitfalls of MUVE learning will be reviewed, with preventive strategies and problem resolutions discussed.

CHAPTER 19

Problems and Pitfalls of MUVE Learning

The purpose of this final "how-to" chapter is to review problems and pitfalls that can occur with MUVE learning activities. Each one is defined and issues related to it are explored, with suggestions for management and prevention.

This chapter is for you if:

1. You are interested in MUVE teaching but concerned about dealing with problems that may come up.

2. You are planning a MUVE learning activity and want to be prepared for potential problems and pitfalls that may arise during the learning activity planning or execution.

3. You have MUVE teaching experience and would like to explore problem prevention strategies.

Learning in virtual space offers great advantages for both students and instructors to explore contextualized learning in a whole new way. As with any teaching method, problems and pitfalls also can arise that should be explored, prevented when possible, and managed when necessary. One of the important keys to MUVE teaching success is an awareness of potential problems and use of preventive strategies to avoid them. Planning a MUVE learning activity should include identification of potential difficulties and implementation of strategies for preventing them. This chapter will outline such potential problems. For each one, case study illustrations are presented along with suggestions for problem prevention and management.

Problems with Technology and Software

Learning activities that utilize computers may provide challenges that should be understood, planned for, and managed effectively so that they do not disrupt the learning process. This can be challenging, but thoughtful prevention and good communication with students is usually all it takes.

Insufficient RAM

Most of the technology problems that accompany MUVE learning activities occur as a result of students' use of computers with limited RAM or use of wireless Internet connections. The requirements for these vary between MUVEs. Most computers currently available to students easily accommodate Second Life® viewer software. Smartphones are not suitable for MUVE learning. Students using very old computers with insufficient RAM may need help finding access to an alternative computer to use for MUVE learning activities. Most campus computer laboratories have computers that accommodate MUVE platform software.

Lag

Lag can be caused by limited band width or RAM, a slow Internet connection, or dense, visually complex MUVE regions. Lag can negatively affect the way the MUVE appears, its visual aspect, and communication in the chat box. Visually, lag manifests as slow resolution of visual aspects of the region. When an avatar first arrives in a region, the environment may be slow to materialize and for a short time appear cloudy or misshapen. The user's avatar body may also be slow to appear. Arrival inworld may be similarly delayed as the avatar body forms. A person experiencing lag may notice that the avatar appears first only as a nebulous cloud or poorly formed shape.

Even a brief momentary lag may be uncomfortable. Generally, the avatar can communicate using the chat box during the lag period ("Don't mind me . . . lag"). At worst, this is distracting for the student who is experiencing the lag and potentially distracting to other students, who may have to talk to a nebulous cloud instead of the human avatar appearance for a short time. If students know this can happen and that it usually resolves quickly, they typically can work around it easily. Note: clothing may also form slowly. The avatar at no time, however, appears nude.

Chat box lag can a bit more challenging. The person experiencing chat box lag may have a delay in the entry of his or her contributions into the chat box. To the other students, this manifests by comments that are delayed or appear out of order in the discussion flow. This is easy to identify in the transcript of the learning activity. Very occasionally, this is serious enough to make student participation too difficult to manage. Most often, however, students can accommodate the nonlinear communication into the discussion.

Loss of Internet Connection

Because many MUVE platforms are based in a software platform outside the user's computer, loss of connection with that platform causes the MUVE world to immediately disappear. The user is immediately logged off. With any loss of Internet connection, even momentary, the user is logged off and his or her avatar disappears. For this reason, students must understand the hazard of using a wireless connection for a MUVE learning activity. If they lose the Internet connection, even for a moment, they will be logged off. They will have to log back on and reengage in the learning activity. The student who is logged off misses part of the activity, and the learning activity is interrupted. These learning activities move quickly, and such loss of time and focus can be very disruptive. If this occurs several times in an activity, the instructor will have to evaluate if the student's participation was sufficient for him or her to receive credit for the activity. If it occurs often across course learning activities, alternative Internet connection options for the student should be discussed. Similarly, an instructor in a MUVE learning activity can absolutely not use a wireless connection, regardless of his or her role or leadership responsibilities. Loss of the activity leader causes a major disruption and should be avoided.

What Is the Fix?

Any course for which MUVE learning activities are planned must have provisions for students who need to use an alternative computer and/or Internet connection if their own cannot support the MUVE learning activity. Issues of fairness and technology access must be addressed so that all participants in the class have access to the technology required to participate in the learning activity. Collaboration with the information technology department is crucial early in the planning process.

Factors related to lag must be repeatedly emphasized in the MUVE orientation. If students understand lag and how it affects the learning activity, they usually take action to prevent it and work around it when it occurs. There is usually minimal negative impact on the learning activity. If students understand, for example, that slow visual resolution is just inconvenient and a bit distracting, they take it in stride. Also, if they know that a peer experiencing lag may have delayed entries, they can accommodate the lag because they know the reason for the delay. In the nonlinear dialogue that can happen in MUVE learning activities, a comment entered in the chat may end with "sorry, lag" to indicate that the student knows his or her entry was delayed. This is the MUVE shorthand for, "I am sorry. I am experiencing some lag and know that this communication is out of place." It is surprising how easily students experienced in social media, in which overlapping and nonlinear communication is commonplace, adapt to this nonlinearity in MUVE learning activity communication. Students are not ever penalized for lag. If students are experiencing severe lag because of limitations in their computer sufficient to cause severe disruption of the learning activity, the instructor can assist the students in identifying an alternative computer or Internet access to use going forward. That said, because there are a variety of reasons why lag occurs, it is often not possible to identify the specific cause of lag.

Loss of Internet connection because a wireless connection is being used can be a potential hazard to MUVE learning activity. This issue should be raised early and often. It is strongly recommended that the no-wireless standard be stated repeatedly, including in the section of the course syllabus where technical requirements for MUVE learning are described. It is recommended that this includes a statement about credit for the learning activity. A student who is repeatedly logged off a learning activity because he or she is using a wireless connection may not expect to receive full credit for the activity. This standard should be clearly addressed in the both the syllabus and the oral orientation.

Firewall Limitations

Occasionally, a school firewall is set up to block certain kinds of software downloads. Simply attempting a download of the MUVE platform software on campus will quickly demonstrate if this is the case. Again, partnering with an information technology specialist is the first step for dealing with this.

Note for Conference Educators: Making conference presentations on MUVE learnng (for example, demonstrating Second Life® in action) can be difficult because most hotels and conference facilities have strict firewall limitations. Presenters beware. Screen shots or videos of the learning activity are preferable.

Issues Related to Student Attitudes

Student attitudes exert a major affect on learning! This is nothing new, but unfamiliar approaches to learning, higher levels of accountability, and greater degrees of learning independence can activate student attitudes that affect their learning—for the better and sometimes for worse. Several particular issues often arise with MUVE learning:

Technology and Learning

Student attitudes toward computer technology and its use in learning vary widely and cannot be assumed on the basis of age, generation, or other demographic factors. Some young students are technology phobic and other, much older students, may be early adopters of technology. Most students currently in undergraduate academic programs grew up with the Internet, are part of the "net generation," and, as digital natives, are assumed to be tech savvy and presumed to be able to adopt new technology easily. Because of their generation's typical activity on social media, they are assumed to be ideal students for learning technology such as MUVEs, but this is not always the case.

Social media communication encourages users to think and act as a group, using crowd sourcing and networking to answer questions and address problems. The instructor considering a MUVE learning activity would do well not to assume that this applies to all students in their class. Unless the students have a documented track record of working effectively with new technology in previous classes, it is a good idea to survey the class. The instructor can use these self-evaluations to generate data about the ease with which students perceive they learn new technologies. The survey can also provide data for the instructor's risk analysis for learning obstacles related to technology. If students perceive that the use of computer technology for learning is challenging for them, that is enough to constitute an obstacle to learning. Repeated offers for one-on-one tutoring and identification of multiple sources of support (instructor, information technology staff, tutorials) are necessary. Sometimes just knowing that there are multiple sources of help gives students the sense of security that enables them to work through a problem independently.

Talking Story: The Class of One

The first class I taught totally in Second Life® was small, only ten students. This was one of the reasons that particular class was chosen for a first all-MUVE class format. Nine of the students had taken a previous class with me in which MUVE technology was used extensively. However, one of the students in the group had no experience in MUVE at all. When I surveyed her attitudes toward learning new technology, however, she had a very positive attitude to computer-based learning and had a "let's do it" attitude toward trying MUVE learning. So although the risk assessment included a high-stakes situation where the consequences for failure would have been very high, there were also very positive factors present. The student new to MUVE had a positive attitude toward learning new technology. In addition, the infectious positive attitude of the rest of the class for MUVE learning provided her, the class of one, a whole team of mentors and tutors.

What Is the Fix?

There is no one size fits all for effective learning. When students have resistance to MUVE learning, it is a good idea to meet with them to explore the resistance. Sometimes just the interest an instructor expresses in such an inquiry is enough for the students to be willing to try MUVE learning. It may be as simple as needing help setting up the MUVE platform software or assistance in getting oriented. The students may already feel insecure about their performance in the class and worried that the new technology will be too much for them. The fix, as much as there is one, is really about listening to the students and attempting to meet them where they are. Problem clarification is the first step. Exploring related issues is the second. Sometimes the problem identified is solvable (additional orientation, skills development). Sometimes an attitude that is causing resistance can be explored together and an agreement reached about how to move forward. In some cases, the student simply may just be asked to jump in and try, with additional instructor check-in and support to follow. Meetings between a student and instructor inworld are often very helpful.

Talking Story: Students with Attitude

One student was struggling with MUVE learning activities ("I can't learn this way"). I offered to meet her inworld to discuss what kind of help she needed. After about twenty minutes together inworld, talking and walking and enjoying the beautiful location I had selected for the meeting, the student reported that the meeting had shown her how easy and effective the MUVE actually was. She even said, "I will keep the transcript of this meeting to help me with the issues we talked about." Another student, who was very tech savvy and had experience with MUVE learning, had a different problem. "Health care is about people so we should learn face-to-face," he said. In this case, I simply asked that he try the learning activity for a few weeks. I explained some of the reasons why I thought it was superior to a face-to-face group for the assignment in question. He remained dubious. After the experience of MUVE learning, he suddenly understood the precise teaching-learning dynamic I had attempted to explain to him. He had seen his peers perform at a level he had never seen before—literally a whole new world opened up for him. He confessed that the experience of MUVE learning had changed his view completely.

When orienting students to MUVE learning, it is a good idea to budget time for one-on-one tutoring if students need it. It is amazing how just a little one-on-one time can make all the difference.

Student Learning Preferences

Student learning preferences also affect the effectiveness of learning activities. Some students prefer independent learning, others prefer a group setting. A MUVE learning activity may trigger—positively or negatively—student preferences. It is interesting to note that while much as this is true, matching student preferences to types of learning activities is not always the solution. I learned this unexpectedly when preparing a course in which MUVE learning activities featured highly.

Talking Story: Not My Cup of Tea?

After an in-class orientation to a mandatory MUVE learning activity, a student whom I knew well from other classes approached me and asked, "Is there another section of this class I could transfer to? I am a read-the-book, take-the-test kind of student, and this class won't work for me." This was an example of a student whose preferred learning style did not match well with MUVE learning. This student taught me a few things about teaching and learning preferences. The bottom line for that student was that he did not want to learn in pairs or groups. He did not want to do self, peer, or group evaluation. He did not want feedback on his behavior or his skills. He wanted to read the book and take the test. Now, I have to say I liked this student a lot and appreciated many things about him, not the least his honesty in stating, in a remarkably uncritical and matter-of-fact way, that my plan for the class did not work for him.

But here is the thing. The health care profession this student was studying for requires one-to-one relationship skills. It is based on group work, team care, and constant quality improvement (self, peer, and group evaluation). This student had a learning preference that had made him successful in the academic (read-the-book, take-the-test) setting but was not a good match for the profession for which he was preparing. When offered a learning activity that went beyond content to skills development and evaluation, this student became uncomfortable. The lesson this student taught me was that while learning preferences are important, they are not the whole story. Sometimes requiring students to move outside their learning style comfort zone is necessary to achieve required learning outcomes.

What Is the Fix?

So the question is not just, "How do you prefer to learn?" any more than an instructor can afford to only ask, "How do I prefer to teach?" Both instructor and student must focus on the performance outcomes that are required. The instructor must design learning activities that fulfill those goals. A master teacher knows that this sometimes means changing teaching methodologies. For students, it may require having to "learn to learn" differently.

When discussing this with students, it is a good idea to identify common goals. For example, "You and I both want you to be successful after you graduate. This will include being effective in therapeutic and team relationships on your clinical unit. Practicing those relationships now will make you more effective in the future." This is one of the ways an instructor can actively support student agency. By identifying performance skills that will be required in the future and offering learning activities that prepare for this performance, the student has a new and effective way to be successful.

Instructor Attitudes

Just as student attitudes can influence the effectiveness of a MUVE learning activity, so also can the attitudes of the instructor. Being honest about one's own attitudes is important when beginning to plan a MUVE learning activity.

Ambiguity Tolerance and Control

It isn't just student attitudes that can be an obstacle to MUVE learning. It is amazing how many buttons can get pushed when an instructor incorporates MUVE learning into his or her pedagogical menu. Even in highly structured, well-organized, and content-heavy MUVE learning activities, the role of student agency and independence is such that the focus is more on student learning than instructor teaching. Although most instructors would say they prefer this (theoretically), once it is real and on the ground, an instructor can experience the shift of focus as overly ambiguous or out of control. Because the focus of MUVE learning is the student experience, the phenomenology of learning differs from traditional learning. Learning activities may not unfold as planned. Flexibility is needed both to support student independence and to maximize learning effectiveness.

What Is the Fix?

Perhaps there is no fix in this case except for the instructor's willingness to be self-reflective, to stay focused on what is working and what needs to be adapted, and to have a singular focus on effective learning. Often in my own MUVE teaching experience, the learning activity that unfolds may be so different from my original conception as to be nearly unrecognizable, but the students are learning like mad! It is often necessary for me to focus on the student learning actually taking place instead of trying to force the activity into its originally intended form.

Teaching in Public: Distractions, Interruptions, Griefing, and Disruptive Students

Unless a learning activity takes place either in a privately run MUVE learning platform or in a private region of a public MUVE such as Second Life®, both instructor and students must adapt to learning in a public environment. Imagine, for example, students doing a small group discussion in a campus cafeteria or dormitory area. Privacy could be difficult to maintain, the group discussion could be overheard, and individuals outside the group could prove disruptive. Distractions posed by people and events in the environment may prove distracting. The same challenges are potentially present when doing MUVE.

There are ways to make a learning activity as private as possible, but the instructor must evaluate and plan for potential problems associated with the public nature of Second Life®. MUVE orientation in must include a discussion with students about the public nature of MUVE learning. Some of the issues that should be discussed include the following:

Privacy

There are several issues related to privacy for MUVE learning activities. Some MUVE learning activities require at least some degree of privacy because of the kind of sharing that takes place in the learning activity. For example, in an ethics discussion group where individuals are sharing personal ethical views and experiences, the risk of being overheard by others outside the group may make it difficult for students to participate comfortably. Dialogue in a chat box in Second Life®, for example, can be overheard the equivalent of thirty (in-world) feet away from the speaker's location. Even a person who passes that close to the learning activity casually, with no intention to disrupt the activity, can read what is being typed in the chat box. They could conceivably also copy what is in the chat box.

Another privacy issue concerns use of transcripts for evaluation of a MUVE learning activity. Transcripts from a learning activity are most often used for evaluation, and for this reason, they are shared with classmates and the instructor. Although these transcripts are not intended for wider distribution, there is no way for an instructor to control inadvertent or intentional misuse or distribution beyond class participants.

What Is the Fix?

There is no way to guarantee privacy in either of the above-mentioned cases. Student orientation to MUVE learning must address this. Students must understand that what they share could potentially be "overheard." Transcripts can be copied by anyone within thirty inworld feet of the "speaker." Student contributions and degree of personal exposure during a learning activity must be moderated in light of this. Respect for each other's privacy and confidentiality in learning activity communication should be discussed. These issues must also be addressed in the syllabus guidelines for MUVE learning activities. If it is desirable to share the transcript of a small group activity with the larger class, deidentification of all the speakers is recommended.

Interruptions

It is a reality of teaching in the public MUVEs that learning activities look interesting to nonstudent residents. Imagine yourself coming upon a group of people engaging in an animated, dynamic conversation about an interesting topic. Wouldn't you want to join in? Even if a discussion group is scheduled for a remote and rarely visited location, nonparticipants occasionally curiously approach the group and ask to join in. Most often, when such individuals are told, "This is a university class. Would you mind honoring our privacy?" they leave, usually with an apology for the inadvertent disturbance. Occasionally, intruders are less respectful, but this is not common. Over the course of five years of supervising hundreds of MUVE learning activities, I can count on one hand the number of times there were disruptive intrusions by people not involved in a learning activity. Only once in my experience did a learning activity have to be stopped and rescheduled for another location and time. For the most part, this kind of interruption is manageable, and students are comfortable requesting privacy and following up as needed with the course instructor. This can be an opportunity for students to use professional behaviors such as limit setting and conflict resolution.

What Is the Fix?

It is important to design learning activities that take place in as private a location as possible. Locations where there is typically a lot of activity are not appropriate for learning activities. That said, student orientation must include guidelines for what to do if a learning activity is interrupted. Usually the reminder, "This is a university class activity. Would you please allow us some privacy?" is all it takes. That said, there are times when it is not, and orientation should also include what to do in the event of serious rudeness, interruption, or other bad behavior on the part of an uninvited avatar. This is called griefing.

Griefing

Sadly, there are Second Life® residents whose idea of fun is being disruptive. These individuals look for gatherings of people for the purpose of disrupting them. For this reason, both instructor and students must know what to do in the event that griefing disrupts a student or learning activity while inworld.

What Is the Fix?

This is another portion of the orientation that should be repeated several times, both in writing and orally. If a griefing event takes place, students should be specifically requested to record the name of the avatar and the time of the griefing event. This is easy to do if a transcript is being kept of the learning activity, as the griefing is recorded in the chat log. If the disruption is temporary or minor enough that the participants can continue the learning activity, the instructor should be notified at the end of the learning activity. If the disruption is serious or for any reason it is not possible to continue the learning activity, students should end the learning activity and notify the instructor. In this case, it may be necessary to reschedule the learning activity. It is important to emphasize to students that if at any time they do not feel comfortable continuing a learning activity because of this kind of intrusion, they should immediately stop the learning activity.

In a case such as this, the instructor should complete a griefing report using the name of the disruptive avatar, the time the event took place, and the nature of the griefing. If needed, a copy of the transcript can be used to document the griefing event. There are consequences for grieving that include loss of privileges and being banned from Second Life®, for example. It is important that students and instructors take these events seriously and follow up with the reporting mechanisms offered. See "Tools to Use" at the end of this chapter for a review of how to report griefing in Second Life®.

Disruptive Students

Occasionally, students who are taking part in the learning activity demonstrate unprofessional or disruptive behavior. Examples include attending a learning activity in an inappropriate avatar form (showing up as a rabbit), wearing inappropriate clothing (a bikini or ball gown), or playing with one's avatar (dancing or other inappropriate physical activity during the learning activity).

What Is the Fix?

Orientation to MUVE learning should include a discussion of professional behavior in MUVE learning. Students should be reminded that professional dress, behavior, and actions are required as much in their avatar form as when they are in class or in a clinical setting. One way to reinforce this is to require a lab coat or other professional attire. Usually a comment to the student before the learning activity begins ("Great outfit . . . but would you please change into something more appropriate for our event tonight?") is sufficient.

Communication Problems

Several communication issues indigenous to the MUVE environment offer unique challenges.

Overlapping Dialogue

Even when there is no lag present, dialogue during the learning activity may be nonlinear. Particularly when dialogue is moving fast, several students are often typing chat entries at the same time. They may hit enter simultaneously, so the dialogue shows up in the chat box in an order that is a little off. The dialogue is not a linear branching from one question to a series of answers but rather a less orderly collection of responses that are slightly out of sequence. Questions and answers may pile up in an odd order. This nonlinearity has been addressed previously. It is awkward but remarkably easy to get used to.

Typing Speed

Chat box entries are typed. Typing speed varies among students. For this reason, the additional time taken by students to add to discussions is much slower than in a face-to-face activity. Surprisingly, these problems do not seem to interfere with the gist of the conversation, but it does take some getting used to. Indeed, slowing down of the discussion speed is one of the things that gives students a chance to think before they speak and to go deeper into the discussion. It would not be surprising for the slowing of communication to be listed as a negative on student learning activity evaluations. In not one of the hundreds of student evaluations I have reviewed, however, has such a criticism been made. Again, it is likely that students who are active in other social media platforms have learned to accommodate nonlinear communication better than those who are not.

Nonverbal Communication

There are only a few nonverbal behaviors Second Life® avatars can make (shrugging, laughing). However, it is interesting to notice how inventive students can be. In the chat dialogue, it is common to see "hahahaha," (joking), (sigh), smiley faces, frown faces, and other ways of indicating nonverbal messages. The instructor can enrich inworld communication by role modeling this kind of "verbal nonverbal" communication.

Benefits of MUVE Communication Limitations

Although the above examples of communication challenges should always be kept in mind, it is also interesting to note that some of the problems that have been mentioned actually offer benefits as well. For example, students for whom English is a second language (ESL) report that group discussions in MUVE chat are easier for them. Typed dialogue comes to them slower, without difficult accents and in visual instead of auditory format. This makes the dialogue easier to translate. They can also type responses without having to worry about pronunciation. Several ESL students have shared that MUVE discussion groups were the first discussion groups in which they participated fully.

The slow speed of interaction that results from typing discussion entries also has a hidden benefit. One of the common things students say about MUVE groups is that, because the speed of interactions is slower with typed dialogue, they have more time to think about what they want to contribute. One of the interesting characteristics of MUVE discussions is that they go deeper faster than face-to-face group discussions. It may be that the slowing of communication actually has a positive impact!

Too Much Change! Too Much Technology! Talking Story: The Class That Went Crazy

In a new program in our school of nursing, learning activities in Second Life® were added to two courses being taught during the first semester of a new program. These activities were wildly unsuccessful in a group that had been assessed to be ideal for MUVE learning. The postactivity assessment concluded that the class was being barraged with new technology throughout the program. The students were having to change and adjust learning skills constantly. The class as a group finally had to confront the well-meaning faculty with the fact that they were inundating the class with both too much change and too much technology.

Well-Intentioned Pedagogical Disasters

Not every experiment works. This is as true for MUVE learning as for any other kind of learning activity. Even a well-planned, well-designed, and well-organized MUVE learning activity with an excellent orientation for a group assessed to be ready may bomb. It is important for the instructor not to blame the technology but rather to understand that new learning activities will include mistakes and unforeseen problems. Instructors should continue to include evaluation of every activity as a way of learning to be a better MUVE instructor. Frank discussions and feedback mechanisms where students can be honest about what worked and what didn't work will not only improve the next MUVE learning activity but also help students learn to improve their own ability to learn from mistakes and misfires.

Tools to Use: How to Report Griefing

Reporting griefing is very easy. On the drop-down menu on the top left of the Second Life® viewer, click on "Help," then "Report Abuse." A screen will come up that prompts the user to indicate the date, time, and other details of the griefing incident. If the abuse was verbal, it can be copied from the learning activity transcript, along with the offending individual's avatar name. This will facilitate the reporting process.

Reader's Roadmap: Where Are We?

The book will now conclude with Chapter 20, which brings it all together with a description of the design and implementation for a course on emotional intelligence, a topic that is particularly effectively when presented in a MUVE learning activity.

CHAPTER 20

Design and Implementation of a MUVE Emotional Intelligence Course

This chapter describes the design and implementation of a course that focuses on the development of emotional intelligence in interdisciplinary teams. This course took place 50 percent in Second Life®, using individual, one-on-one, and small group learning activities.

This chapter is for you if:

1. You are interested in how a complex topic like emotional intelligence can be addressed using MUVE learning.

2. You are interested in how MUVE learning can be developed as a core teaching methodology.

Introduction and Purpose

Emotional intelligence (EI) is a concept that has evolved over the past twenty years as ideas about intelligence have changed. A combination of inter- and intra-personal intelligences as described by Howard Gardner's theory of multiple intelligences, EI is now understood to be an important factor in organizational behavior, performance evaluation, and leadership effectiveness. Hundreds of research studies across dozens of professional disciplines and many countries have provided evidence for the relationship between EI ability and important organizational outcomes. These outcomes include performance in the work-place, retention on the job, prosocial organizational behaviors, employee health, team effectiveness, positive conflict styles, and numerous measures of leadership effectiveness.

As an emotional intelligence researcher whose work focuses on workplace performance, I knew there would come a time when I would be asked to make suggestions on how to teach and improve EI abilities. Although modalities such as peer coaching, mentoring, and didactic presentations have been described in the research literature, I felt confident that MUVE learning was a good peda-gogical match with learning and improving EI ability. Serendipitously, as I was coming to this conclusion, I was asked to teach an undergraduate course for the honors department at the University of Hawai'i. I chose as the topic for the course "Developing Emotional Intelligence in Interdisciplinary Teams." The course was designed to be taught at least 50 percent in a MUVE. In the course, solo, one-on-one, and small group MUVE learning activities were used to help students learn about the various EI models, to identify their own EI abilities and areas for growth, and to practice EI skills needed for effective one-on-one and team performance.

This chapter will use the previously described checklist for planning a MUVE learning activity to describe the assessment, planning, implementation, and evaluation that took place for the course.

Assessment of Instructor Strengths/Weaknesses

By the time I was planning the course, I had planned, executed, and evaluated hundreds of MUVE learning activities. Although motivated to continuously develop my MUVE teaching ability, I considered myself an expert in MUVE teaching. I had completed several research studies on learning outcomes for MUVE learning and presented several conference workshops on the subject. My confidence and skill level were both high. I was also very excited that my two areas of interest, EI and MUVE learning, were coming together. My motivation and excitement level were very high.

My self-assessment included a few potential obstacles. This course involved a younger learner population than I was accustomed to and one outside my own professional discipline. Another potential weak area was IT support. Because the class was outside my own department, the IT team that had supported my MUVE teaching so far would not be available to course participants. I would be assuming both instructor and IT support roles for the course.

Summary Evaluation: On the whole, I assessed that instructor strengths outweighed instructor weaknesses for the planned MUVE-focused course.

Assessment of the Target Student Population's Strengths/Weaknesses

The proposed EI course was an elective course, and students had access to the course syllabus prior to registering for the course. This ensured that students understood that the MUVE was a major modality for learning in the course. In addition, they understood computer requirements and the opportunity for solo, one-on-one, and small group learning. Students would be literally signing up for this kind of learning. It was even possible that MUVE learning was a draw for some students' selection of the course. At the least, students who registered for the class were open to MUVE learning. It was not likely that any student with major resistance to MUVE learning would select the course. On the positive side, MUVE learning is often energizing and interesting to students, and this energy often helps students get over unanticipated obstacles.

The student readiness assessment included several weak areas as well. Students would be from disciplines outside my own and also would be younger and less academically experienced than the students I usually taught. Although it was likely that the students had heard about MUVEs, it was not likely that they had been involved with MUVE learning. They would also be freshman and sophomore students, relatively inexperienced academically.

Summary Evaluation: Although there were both strengths and weaknesses represented in the prospective student course participants, on the whole, positive student factors were assessed to outweigh negative ones.

Technology Support

The university IT department was experienced with MUVE learning and had supported several university departments with its implementation. There were no problems with the university firewall, and there were several places on campus where the MUVE platform I had chosen was installed on computers that were available to students. Numerous courses, including ones taught totally in a MUVE setting, had been taught without major problems. However, there was no single IT staff member who was responsible for student MUVE problems. If I wanted continuity in problem solving, it was likely that I would be responsible for much of the technology problem solving one-on-one with my students.

Summary Evaluation: Although there were significant positive factors related to technology support, in my assessment, I flagged technology as a potential challenge for the course.

Would the Course Use Simple or Complex Learning Activities?

The design of the course enabled me to begin with very simple MUVE learning activities and progress to more complex ones. I formulated a plan for developing MUVE learning skills gradually as the course progressed. The course would use both simple, unstructured learning activities and very complex, structured ones. This plan matched the pedagogical goals for the course as well, as simple concepts were developed to provide a foundation for more complex ones.

Simple, relatively unstructured learning activities were used throughout the course. In the beginning, these activities enabled students to build on their MUVE orientation and experience a simple set of learning goals in a solo activity. Later, more difficult topics were addressed using simple and relatively unstructured activities. An example of a simple, unstructured assignment used to build MUVE skills was the first learning activity for the course. In this solo learning activity, students simply went to any MUVE region and explored the region for thirty minutes. During their exploration, they were asked to make a list of descriptors for what MUVE learning was like. At the end of the time inworld, they were asked to review their list and to think about what MUVE learning would be like, including the advantages and disadvantages they anticipated.

Another learning activity used later in the course involved students observing the behavior of the MUVE residents and attempting to identify emotional intelligence abilities that were illustrated in the interactions they observed. In addition, students were asked to identify interactions in which EI abilities were not used and the interactional consequences that resulted. (See Appendix 29 for a description of the learning activity and its evaluation matrix.)

One-on-one MUVE learning activities were also used throughout the course. The first one-on-one learning activity involved "getting to know you" exercises in which student pairs met to discuss their ideas about the nature of consciousness, intelligence, and the theory of multiple intelligences applied to them. Later in the course, a one-on-one learning activity was used for students to practice feedback skills and validation of their self and group evaluations. In the final weeks of the course, students used one-one-one activities to discuss their ideas about MUVE learning and the advantages and disadvantages MUVE learning they had experienced in their own learning. An example of a more complex, one-on-one learning activity that was scheduled for later in the course was the Rewriting History learning activity previously described.

Small group learning was also used throughout the course. In the beginning, simple small group discussions about intelligence, multiple intelligences, and emotional intelligence supported the students' exploration of these concepts. In a learning activity called Quest 2, they demonstrated emotional intelligence abilities and collected data on EI abilities demonstrated by the group (see Appendix 32 for the activity description and Appendix 33 for the list of EI abilities and their operational definitions used for the activity).

Later, more sophisticated small group teamwork assignments were assigned, such as the collaboration assignment presented previously in this text. A very complex leadership evaluation activity was planned for the later part of the course. In that activity, a small group of students went on a quest in a specific MUVE region. In this place, the group had to locate certain items and perform group tasks within specific limitations. Group members took turns being group leader. A leadership evaluation tool was used after the hour-long activity to evaluate the effectiveness of group leadership throughout the quest. Another complex activity involved the collection and analysis of data on emotional intelligence on the basis of public observations. (See Appendix 30 and Appendix 31 for the data evaluation grid and assignment description for the paper that was assigned for this activity.)

Summary Evaluation: The combination of simple and complex learning activities matched well with the planned course.

Should the Course Use Optional or Mandatory Learning Activities?

Because MUVE learning constituted a primary learning methodology for the course, the MUVE learning activities for the course were mandatory. I ensured that there was sufficient experience in MUVE learning early in the course so that students who found that they did not want to participate in this kind of learning could drop the course if they preferred to. In my experience teaching this course, no student has chosen to drop the course.

Learning Activities and Performance Outcomes: Planning and Evaluation

As the syllabus for the course was written, specific learning objectives were matched with planned MUVE learning activities and specific performance outcomes. An evaluation matrix for each learning activity was devised based on the learning objectives and specific performance outcomes for each. A brief description of each learning activity was written for distribution to students that included the way evaluation would be accomplished for the activity. The steps for involvement in the learning activity were clearly outlined and expectations of student performance clearly stated. The grading matrix for each activity was attached to each learning activity description. Responsibilities for self-evaluation, peer evaluation, and/or group evaluation were also included.

Because the course was a new one, I took care to include careful summative and formative evaluation for both the individual course activities and the overall course itself. This not only helped me to improve the course activities and the course itself but also enabled me to quantify the effectiveness of MUVE learning for this particular subject.

Course Syllabus

The course syllabus was written to include a general description of MUVE learning, the tech requirements needed to support the MUVE learning, and brief descriptions of each MUVE learning activity included in the course. The technology description included a discussion of the importance of not using wireless Internet access during MUVE learning activities and the availability of alternate computer access.

MUVE Regions Used in the Course

Because a wide range of solo, one-on-one, and small group MUVE learning activities was used for this course, a wide variety of MUVE locations was used. Small group activities took place in intimate settings that fostered good conversations. Team exercises such as quests and leadership activities took place in specialized settings that provided meaningful contexts for the learning activities. In the early part of the course, specific locations were assigned for learning activities. Later in the course, students were permitted to select locations for many of the activities.

Orientation to MUVE Learning, Second Life®, and Individual Learning Activities

A spiraled orientation to MUVE learning, the specific MUVE used, and individual learning activities was planned. After an initial assessment of the class's computer and technology skills, MUVE learning was presented in a face-to-face class. This presentation included a demonstration of Second Life® projected into the classroom. All students had an opportunity to operate an avatar that was being used for demonstration purposes. They were able to experience through this hands-on experience how easy MUVE learning can be. This class activity was followed by the students' independent self-guided orientation to Second Life®. Key points were again reviewed in class the following week. Problems and obstacles were discussed, and when needed, students received individual assistance from the course instructor. Orientation materials and background information such as an article that discussed MUVE learning were included on the course website. Based on students' report after orientation was completed, MUVE orientation took on the average less than two hours. The most common difficulty that students reported was minor difficulty learning avatar navigation. Patience with the learning curve was required. At each face-to-face class, some aspect of MUVE learning was discussed and important concepts such as avoiding wireless Internet access were emphasized. Orientation information was reviewed repeatedly, particularly during the first weeks of the course.

Avatar Names and Sign-up Procedures

Students received both in-person and hard-copy orientation to creation of their avatar, including naming procedures, appearance, and professionalism issues. Several students required reinforcement of this material when inappropriate names or avatar appearance were used. Several duplicate names required alternative naming procedures. A procedure for students to sign up for small group activities was made using the course web page's discussion function.

Evaluation of MUVE Learning in the Course

Approximately a dozen learning activities were used in the Emotional Intelligence MUVE course. Several aspects of the MUVE learning were particularly striking. First, I observed that the MUVE activities gave students an opportunity to use what they had learned from assigned reading and class lectures. I also noticed that the sophistication of evaluation methods made possible by MUVE learning made behavior change and skills development a strong component of the course. This offered the course benefits similar to those using simulation or clinical practica, with the added benefit of transcript use for evaluation. Students came away from the course with a level of mastery that would not have been possible in a traditional course. Student satisfaction with the course was high. Evaluation metrics reflected this quantitatively, as did anecdotal comments added to the course evaluation. Instructor satisfaction was also high, primarily because of the high degree of actual performance evaluation that the MUVE learning activities made possible.

This course illustrated the way that MUVE learning enhances engagement of content material that focuses on students' behaviors and the development of skills, not simply factual or conceptual engagement with course material. In this respect, the course showcased the pedagogical advantages of MUVE learning to both instructor and students. In addition, the course also illustrated the way the best practices outlined in this text can be easily applied to enrich and expand courses taught with traditional methodologies. The result was an innovative approach to teaching and learning that took learning to a new level for students and instructors alike.

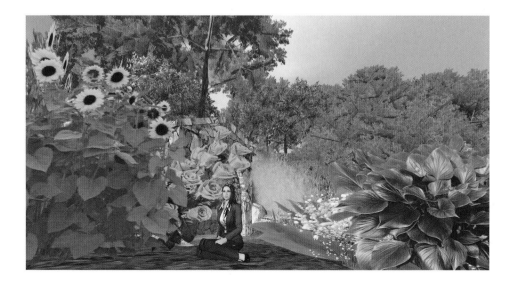

PART IV

Appendixes

APPENDIX 1

Eight Characteristics of a Third Place

- Neutral ground—without political, social, or economic charges
- Leveling—everyone is the same; there are no prerequisites to being there nor social levels of those who attend
- Needs met easily and intentionally
- "The regulars"—people make it "their place" and go there regularly
- Grounded, humble feeling without showiness or pretense
- A playful mood pervades
- A homelike feeling
- Conversation is the main activity

APPENDIX 2

Grading Rubric Template for a Clinic Patient Interview Assignment

Objective	Specific Data	Met Outcome	Comments
Objective 1: The student will be able to identify the critical targeted assessment elements of the disease pathology in the courses of the patient interview either as nurse (elicits the information) or the patient (presents the information)		YES: NO:	
Objective 2: The student will be able to list differential diagnoses and to identify the rationale for the selected diagnosis		YES: NO:	
Objective 3: The student will be able to identify the critical labs and diagnostics related to the presented pathology (the patient includes pertinent labs in the presentation of the illness; the nurse is able to identify the labs pertinent to the disease)		YES: NO:	
Objective 4: The student will be able to identify specific interventions to be included in the initial treatment of the presented pathology (nurse participant only)		YES: NO:	
Objective 5: The student will be able to identify and communicate to the patient the diagnosis for which he or she is being treated	The nurse will explain the disease and diagnostic	YES: NO:	

(continued)

Objective	Specific Data	Met Outcome	Comments
and to explain the treatment and its complications	follow-up required for treatment and pharmacological and other treatments indicated by their disease presentation		
Objective 6: The student will, on the basis of the patient interview, develop a plan of care that is appropriate for the patient and disease		YES: NO:	
Objective 7: The student will, on the basis of the patient interview, develop a teaching plan that is appropriate for the patient and disease		YES: NO:	
Total grade:			

APPENDIX 3

Sample Learning Activity 12: Mock Job Interview

Introduction: This is a one-on-one MUVE learning activity that gives participants an opportunity to role-play job interviews, get feedback on their performance and suggestions for improvement, and have the opportunity to repeat the assignment and implement new behaviors.

Learning Activity Goal: The purpose of this learning activity is to simulate a job interview and to offer an opportunity for performance review, feedback, and skills improvement.

Performance Outcomes: By the end of the thirty-minute learning activity and its evaluation, the participants will:

1. Complete a mock job interview.

2. Describe the strengths and weaknesses of their performance during the mock interview.

3. Identify and describe the obstacles they experienced that affected their ability to interview effectively.

4. Identify what behaviors they would do differently in a subsequent interview.

MUVE Setup Requirements and Activity Procedures

Setup: No specific setup is required for this learning activity other than the identification of locations the students can choose from to conduct their interviews in an office environment such as a nurse manager or personnel officer would use. Students acting in the role of the interviewer should be provided a list of questions to ask the person being interviewed.

Activity Procedures:

1. Students doing this assignment should be assigned pairs. One student will act as the interviewing nurse; the other student will be the interviewer.

2. The student acting as the interviewer will use a script of questions provided by the instructor for use during the interview.

3. Both participants should stay "in role," including social interactions before and after the interview. This should include greetings outside the interview area, ending the interview and leaving, and so on.

4. At the end of the twenty-minute interview, participants will leave the interview room and for the remaining ten minutes share their perceptions of the interview, both what they think went well and suggestions for improvement.

Evaluation

Participants will summarize the strengths and weaknesses of their partner interviewer and forward it to the instructor along with the exercise transcript. The instructor will review the transcript and forward the grade (if the assignment is graded) and additional comments to each participant. If a portfolio is used for the course, the packet of transcript, evaluation summary, and instructor feedback and, if appropriate, the grade should be included.

Instructional Notes: This learning activity is particularly effective when preceded by didactic presentations of interviewing strategy, discussion of appearance, nonverbal communication, and self-management of anxiety. Several different sets of interview questions should be available to students for use when they reverse roles.

APPENDIX 4

Summative Evaluations for MUVE Learning Activities

Evaluation Grid for Individual MUVE Learning Activities

MUVE Learning Activity: _____   Semester: _____   Year: _____

Criteria	Month 1	Month 2	Month 3	Month 4	Month 5	Month Average
Percentage of students who met 100 percent of learning objectives for the semester						
Percentage of students who met > 80 percent of learning objectives for the semester						
Percentage of students who met > 70 percent of learning objectives for the semester						
Percentage of students who met < 70 percent of learning objectives for the semester						
Percentage of groups that met small group learning objectives (passing grade)						

APPENDIX 5

Tracking Student Performance over Time

Student: _____

Learning Activity Date	Percentage of Content Objectives Met	Percentage of IPR Objectives Met	Percentage of Team Objectives Met	Comments (Changes in Behaviors Targeted for Improvement)

Summary Comments:

Insert graphic representation of data above:

APPENDIX 6

Student Self-Evaluation Rubric
for Ethics Small Group Discussion

Student:_____

Objective	Possible Points	Points Achieved	Suggestions for Improvement
1. Identification of the ethical principles (autonomy, fidelity, beneficence, nonmaleficence, paternalism) illustrated in the ethical dilemma under discussion	20		
2. Identification of the ethical principle that most describes students' personal view of the ethical dilemma under discussion	20		
3. Contribution of an approximately equal number of comments to the discussion as other participants	10		
4. Responds to peers during the discussion at least once (agreeing, disagreeing, affirming, inviting further discussion of a subject)	15		
5. Participation in formulation of a consensus statement for the questions posed in the discussion group assignments	15		
*Leader: welcome students, start the group on time, state			*For group leader only: A leader

(continued)

Objective	Possible Points	Points Achieved	Suggestions for Improvement
the group task, facilitate the group discussion, assist the group with staying on task, serve as timekeeper, end the discussion on time, and distribute transcript			may get 5 points for leading the group and may have a total score of 105 percent
Self-evaluation	5		
Peer evaluation (your evaluation of a peer)	5		
Group evaluation	5		
Total assignment score (includes strength and weakness data listed below)	100		

Performance Improvement Planning (5 points):

What was your greatest area of strength in this assignment?

Was there anything you had planned to follow up on from a previous assignment in this one? (Performance improvement plans?)

What was your greatest area of weakness?

What would you like to do differently next time?

APPENDIX 7

Peer Evaluation for Ethics Small Group Discussion

Student being evaluated: _____   Student doing the evaluation: _____

Objective	Possible Points	Points Achieved	Comments/ Suggestions for Improvement
1. Identification of the ethical principles (autonomy, fidelity, beneficence, nonmaleficence, paternalism) illustrated in the ethical dilemma under discussion	20		
2. Identification of the ethical principle that most describes the peer's personal view of the ethical dilemma under discussion	20		
3. Contribution of an approximately equal number of comments to the discussion as other participants	20		
4. Responds to peers during the discussion at least once (agreeing, disagreeing, affirming, requesting an expansion of or query about their statement, etc.)	20		
5. Participation in formulation of a consensus statement for the questions posed in the discussion group assignments	20		
Total assignment score	100		

What do you think your peer's greatest strength was? Is there an area for which you would suggest improvement?

APPENDIX 8

Group Evaluation for Ethics Small Group Discussion

Group being evaluated: _____   Student doing the evaluation: _____

Objective	Possible Points	Points Achieved	Comments/ Suggestions for Improvement
1. Identification of the ethical principles (autonomy, fidelity, beneficence, nonmaleficence, paternalism) illustrated in the ethical dilemma under discussion	20		
2. Identification of the ethical principle that most describes students' personal view of the ethical dilemma under discussion	20		
3. Contribution of an approximately equal number of comments among participants	20		
4. Responds to peers during the discussion at least once (agreeing, disagreeing, affirming, requesting an expansion of or query about their statement, etc.): 5 total for group	20		
5. Participation in formulation of a consensus statement for the questions posed in the discussion group assignments	20		
Total assignment score	100		

Summary of group strength and areas suggested for development:

APPENDIX 9

Instructor Summary for Individual Students: Ethics Small Group Discussion

Student being evaluated: _____ Peer evaluation by: _____

Peer evaluation completed on: _____

Objective	Possible Points	Self-Evaluation Score	Peer Evaluation Score	Instructor Evaluation Score	Average Total Score
1. Identification of the ethical principles (autonomy, fidelity, beneficence, nonmaleficence, paternalism) illustrated in the ethical dilemma under discussion	20				
2. Identification of the ethical principle that most describes their own personal view of the ethical dilemma under discussion	15				
3. Contribution of an approximately equal number of comments to the discussion as other participants	10				
4. Responds to peers during the discussion at least once (agreeing, disagreeing, affirming, requesting an expansion of or query about their statement, etc.)	15				

(continued)

Objective	Possible Points	Self-Evaluation Score	Peer Evaluation Score	Instructor Evaluation Score	Average Total Score
5. Participation in formulation of a consensus statement for the questions posed in the discussion group assignments	20				
Self-evaluation completed	5				
Group evaluation completed	5				
Peer evaluation completed	5				
Total assignment score	100				

Summary of student strengths/weaknesses and suggestions for improvement:

APPENDIX 10

Grading Rubric: Genetics Discussion Group

Objective	Possible Points	Points Awarded	Comments and Suggestions for Improvement
1. Identify chromosomal abnormalities associated with five common diseases	20		
2. Describe eight types of genetic disease transmission	20		
3. Analyze characteristics of progeny anticipated from a series of crosses of dominant and recessive genes	20		
4. Describe the genetic phenomena of antibiotic resistance and explain why completion of a prescribed antibiotic regimen is important for antibiotic resistance prevention	20		
Self-evaluation	5		
Group evaluation	5		
Total assignment score	100		

APPENDIX 11

Grading Rubric: Small Group Learning Activity for Disabilities

Objective	Possible Points	Points Earned	Comments and Suggestions for Improvement
1. Definition and description of three kinds of access barriers for people with physical disabilities	12		
2. Definition and description of cognitive disability	4		
3. Definition and description of cognitive disabilities (minimum 2)	8		
4. Definition and description of neurological disability	4		
5. Definition and description of neurological disabilities (minimum 3)	12		
6. Definition and description of auditory disability	4		
7. Definition and description of auditory disabilities (minimum 2)	8		
8. Definition and description of two strategies for working with auditory disabilities	8		
9. Definition and description of speech disability	4		
10. Definition and description of speech disabilities (minimum 2)	8		

(continued)

Objective	Possible Points	Points Earned	Comments and Suggestions for Improvement
11. Two strategies for working with speech disabilities	4		
12. Identification of issues related to public image of people with disabilities (minimum 2)	8		
13. Identify terms that can be used to describe those who are disabled	4		
Self-evaluation	6		
Group evaluation	6		
Total assignment score	100		

APPENDIX 12

Sample Learning Activity 9: Clinical Rounds for Systemic Lupus Erythematosus (SLE)

Objective	Course Content Applied	Suggested Leader Questions	Evaluation
1. The student participant will demonstrate integration of course content during group discussion in Second Life®.	Course content from N613: —Pathophysiology —Phenomena of autoimmunity —Concept of self/nonself —What sets off SLE flares —Use of steroids for SLE, including complications of tapering —How to live with SLE —Complications of SLE —p/s issues R/t SLE	1. What causes SLE? 2. What is autoimmunity? 3. What happens when the body ID's a body cell as NONSELF? 4. What do you think happens when the kidneys and other organ systems are full of these huge antigen/antibody complexes? 5. What causes SLE flares and what is the physiological connection?	Participant #1: ___ Participant #2: ___ Participant #3: ___ Participant #4: ___ Participant #5: ___ Participant #6: ___ Participant #7: ___
2. The student participant will demonstrate team participation.	—Everyone will participate —Each student will learn from the others: each student will respond positively, negatively, or cumulatively to at least one other student during clinical rounds		Participant #1: ___ Participant #2: ___ Participant #3: ___ Participant #4: ___ Participant #5: ___ Participant #6: ___ Participant #7: ___

(continued)

Objective	Course Content Applied	Suggested Leader Questions	Evaluation
3. The student participant will demonstrate novice skills of multidisciplinary teamwork.	—IPR behaviors r/t effective team behavior —Not interrupting —Following up on each other's comments (–/+feedback) —Ability to summarize what they learned	What is one take-home piece that you got from this clinical rounds today?	Participant #1: ___ Participant #2: ___ Participant #3: ___ Participant #4: ___ Participant #5: ___ Participant #6: ___ Participant #7: ___
4. The student participant will demonstrate novice role development skills.	Each student will be able to demonstrate clinical prioritization skills	As an NP, what would your priorities for this patient's care be? What will you keep in mind for future visits?	Participant #1: ___ Participant #2: ___ Participant #3: ___ Participant #4: ___ Participant #5: ___ Participant #6: ___ Participant #7: ___

APPENDIX 13

Clinical Rounds Learning Activity Description

The goals of the clinical rounds assignment is to:

1. Apply the content covered in the text each week to a simulated clinical situation.

2. Integrate the physiological, psychological, and pathophysiological concepts represented by the patient scenarios into an understanding of the patient's condition and a plan for his or her care.

3. Utilize collaboration in the clinical rounds team to problem solve and integrate course concept within the context of a team.

4. Develop leadership skills across the semester, with a goal of each student leading clinical rounds twice in the semester, as well as performing the role of clinical rounds evaluator and also serving as the "patient" in clinical rounds.

The procedure for the clinical rounds assignment is as follows:

1. Each week, the discussion group members will identify a day and time for clinical rounds to take place. The roles of leader, evaluator, and patient will be assigned by the group.

2. On the syllabus weekly content description, each week general topics for the clinical rounds assignment are identified in the color designated for the discussion group on the syllabus schedule.

3. The clinical rounds group members are responsible for reading relevant material in the course text, to include the following: a review of normal anatomy and physiology if needed, review and summary of the pathophysiology of the illness/illnesses to be covered in clinical rounds, risk factors associated with the condition, expected changes in the review of systems, associated diagnostic tests and labs, typical treatments/procedures associated with the condition, and prognosis

with and without treatment. A worksheet may be found in the course materials (Modules section, course website) that may be of assistance in preparing for clinical rounds.

4. The group will meet in Second Life® (Second Health Hospital, Poly clinic landing area) for 30 to 45 minutes to complete the clinical rounds assignment. The clinical rounds leader first welcomes the group and leads the group to an area just outside the patient's area. In the first 10 minutes, the leader introduces the group to the pathology the patient has and the group briefly reviews the most important elements of the illness. Areas of possible priority to bring up with the patient are reviewed. The group then goes into the patient area, greets the patient, and asks a series of questions about the patient's experience of illness. THIS IS NOT A FULL H&P. If the group has questions about VS, labs, etc., they can ask the instructor at this time, but the general focus is on the patient's experience. After 10 minutes, the group leaves and the leader then leads a discussion about priorities for the patient, issues that will need to be discussed, or specific problems that have been already identified. For the final few minutes, the group leaves the clinical area and does a few minutes of postconference. "What was your take-home piece today?" An evaluation of how the group did as a "group brain" will also be reviewed. The dialogue in the chat box will be highlighted and copied, then pasted into a Word file and forwarded to the instructor. The group evaluator will provide the instructor with an evaluation of the clinical rounds (using the clinical rounds prep sheet and the evaluation of the participation of group members).

5. The clinical rounds leader will copy the dialogue from the activity and forward it to the course instructor for review.

Evaluation of the clinical rounds assignment: Student participation in clinical rounds is expected to reflect their knowledge and understanding of the patient and their condition. Grading is according to the participation rubric.

APPENDIX 14

Sample Dialogue from the First Third of Clinical Rounds

For this activity, the group meets at the Second Life® landing area for the Second Health PolyClinic. After everyone has arrived, the group enters the hospital together and enters a clinical practice area, specifically a Medical-Surgical Clinic. Entering the clinic, the group starts the first third of the clinical rounds just outside the door of the examination room where the patient is waiting.

Group leader: Our patient today has SLE . . . we are talking about it because it does have a skin manifestation . . . but we will be really talking about it next week . . . as it is an immune problem . . . anyone want to say something about what causes SLE?

Student 1: It is a dysfunction of the immune system.

Student 2: The body attacks itself.

Student 3: Right . . . autoimmunity!

Group leader: Anyone want to take a stab at defining autoimmunity?

Student 2: The body does not recognize its own cells.

Student 1: Right—they confuse a normal cell with an invading organism! (they don't tell you that in A&P class) . . . and in autoimmunity, the ID badge doesn't work! So "self cells" are identified as invaders!

Student 4: That is gross . . . imagine your body not being able to recognize itself!

Group leader: I agree . . . in the case of SLE . . . part of what the body doesn't recognize is its own genetic material! YUK!

Student 3: It is kinda like being "allergic" to YOURSELF! The idea has always weirded me out . . . hahahah.

Student 4: So this is what they call self versus nonself.

Group leader: Right. So . . . what happens when the body id's something as NONSELF?

Student 1: The body immune cells attack it.

Student 4: What she said is exactly right . . . right, the cells all gang up and destroy the "nonself."

Group leader: This is how I remember it . . . one cell HUGS the antigen then another covers it with chocolate sauce! This makes it desirable to eat . . .

Student 4: I remember that part. The antibodies and other cells hold onto it tight . . . that makes this huge antigen-antibody complex.

Group leader: Right! Then . . . (here is where the chocolate sauce comes in) . . . other parts of the immune system are attracted to it and EAT it . . . so here is the thing . . . suddenly, you have all these HUGE antigen-antibody complexes EVERYWHERE. So what do you think happens when suddenly the kidneys are full of them?

Student 4: Damage to the kidney . . . and any other organ where the antigen-antibody complexes junk up the body's tissues.

Group leader: The kidneys are among our most sensitive cells . . . but you can have a TON of damage before the BUN and creatinine start to rise. How would this affect other organs?—how about the heart? . . . So what about the lungs? What would all that junk do in the lungs? how about the brain?

Student 1: Well, SLE patients have dysrhythmias . . . that could be one effect on the heart.

Student 2: Right . . . and there are lung diseases associated with SLE . . . and neurological changes are common.

Group leader: OK . . . the physiology is fascinating and we could talk about it all clinical rounds, but let's go back to what can set off a SLE flare . . . any ideas?

Student 3: Sun will do it.

Student 4: Right . . . and stress.

Group leader: Right . . . lots of things that affect how these patients live . . . so SLE is a GREAT nursing disease . . . these patients really need a great nurse! (we know about stress) . . . OK . . . let's go talk with our patient . . . remember, not a full interview or H&P . . . just talk story a bit . . .

This beginning third of the clinical rounds exercise takes about 10 minutes and transitions into the second third, where students talk with the patient. The group moves together into the examination room to meet the patient.

APPENDIX 15

Sample Dialogue from the Second Third of Clinical Rounds

This second third of the clinical rounds learning activity takes place in the clinic examination room.

Group leader: (leads the group into the patient's room)

Group leader: Hi, Mrs. Smith, here are the nursing students I told you about. Thank you for agreeing to speak with them. Is this still a good time?

Patient: Yes, thanks for coming to talk with me.

Student 1: Mrs. Smith, I know you are a nursing student and that the SLE diagnosis is new for you. Do you know much about SLE?

Patient: I feel like I should, being a nursing student, but honestly I don't remember much and haven't had time to research it, so I really don't know much.

Student 2: So it sounds like learning about SLE will be pretty important.

Patient: Oh, YES! I could use some help with that . . . I am kinda stressed by this whole thing and I don't know where to begin.

Student 3: What has been the hardest part of the symptoms for you?

Patient: Well, I have to say, the fatigue has been awful. I just can't do much and with school, and work, and my kids, I just can't keep up.

Student 4: I am not sure I could keep up with all that (laughing).

Patient: (sniffles) I feel a little teary . . . I feel like I should, but honestly, I just can't any more . . . and I am worried about what kind of mother I will be if I am sick all the time.

Student 2: It sounds like you are trying hard to do well at a lot of things . . .

Student 4: It would be hard for a healthy person to keep up with all that!

Patient: It is true . . . people always say I expect too much.

Student 1: Going back to your diagnosis, what got you to the doctor.

Patient: Well it is this darned rash . . . it looks so ugly, doesn't it . . . and then he did some tests and my anti-DNA antibodies came back positive.

Student 4: Were blood tests done to evaluate your kidneys?

Patient: Yes, so far so good, thankfully.

Group leader: There are lots more things we would like to ask you, Mrs. Smith, but we have run out of time . . . thanks for your time.

Student 1: Yes, thank you!

Student 3: Bye, Mrs. Smith.

Patient: Goodbye, thanks for your time.

This second third of the clinical rounds exercise takes about 10 minutes and transitions into the third, where students leave the patient, depart from the examination room, and return to the private area in the clinic where they can discuss what they learned from the patient and how it applies to the disease they are focusing on.

APPENDIX 16

Sample Dialogue from the Last Third of Clinical Rounds

The group has returned to the hall outside the examination room.

Group leader: So, what do you all think about our patient today?

Student 1: Wow, what an awful disease.

Student 2: I was thinking that she has a lot of the really hard aspects of the disease.

Group leader: Can you say some more?

Student 2: The fatigue is really hard under the best of circumstances, and she is so busy!

Student 4: She really is going to have to let go of some of this . . .

Group leader: What are the symptoms you heard about that are classic for SLE?

Student 2: The rash . . . a butterfly rash on the face.

Student 4: The fatigue . . . especially the way it comes and goes episodically is classic.

Group leader: Right . . . in terms of the plan of care, where will you begin?

Student 1: The patient education is going to be a high priority.

Student 4: Right . . . she is intelligent and really motivated, so teaching her should be a first step.

Student 2: I am really worried about her expectations of herself . . . she wants to be able to do everything.

Student 4: Also her self-image . . . she is hard on herself . . . and grieving the changes in her appearance.

Group leader: I am hearing a common denominator there . . . anyone else hear it?

Student 3: STRESS!!!

Group leader: Hahahah . . . right, and we all know how easy that is to deal with that.

Student 1: So stress management will be huge.

Group leader: What else?

Student 2: Well, I was thinking living here in Hawaii is going to be tough in terms of sun exposure, and her rash may be related to that.

Group leader: So it sounds like we have a lot to think about . . . and lots more to talk about. Our time is nearly up, what is one take home piece you have picked up today?

Student 1: I was thinking the fatigue so many students have really make SLE a problem for students.

Student 3: I was realizing how many systems are affected . . . I always think of the skin and forget the other system effects.

Student 4: For me, it is those antigen-antibody complexes . . . thinking about the micropathology helps me understand why so many other tissues are involved.

Group leader: These are all good . . . let's step out of the clinic for a minute now for a quickie post conference.

During the final minutes of the exercise, students share their reflections on how the group performed and what they learned from the activity.

APPENDIX 17

Clinical Rounds: Summative Evaluation

Number of student participants:

Entries per participant

Participant #	Entries
1	
2	
3	
4	
5	
6	

Average entries per participant

Number of participants with at least five entries

Content Objective:

Did the participant demonstrate integration of course content during group discussion?

Participant #	Yes/No
1	
2	
3	
4	
5	
6	

Did the participant demonstrate understanding of the focus pathology during group discussion?

Participant #	Yes/No
1	
2	
3	
4	
5	
6	

Number of students meeting content objective

Process objective:

Did the participant demonstrate team interaction?

Participant #	Yes/No
1	
2	
3	
4	
5	
6	

Did the participant demonstrate novice role development?

Participant #	Yes/No
1	
2	
3	
4	
5	
6	

Number of students meeting process objective

(Attach dialogue to this form)

APPENDIX 18

Tracking Student Performance over Time

Student: _____

Learning Activity Date	Percentage of Content Objectives Met	Percentage of IPR Objectives Met	Percentage of Team Objectives Met	Comments: (Changes in Behaviors Targeted for Improvement)

Insert graphic representation of data above:

Comments:

APPENDIX 19

Grading Rubric for Clinical Rounds Learning Activity 14: Asthma

Date: _____   Group: _____

Student 1: _____   Student 2: _____   Student 3: _____

Student 4: _____   Student 5: _____   Student 6: _____

Student leader, if utilized: _____   Student in patient role, if utilized: _____

Objectives	Outcomes	Course Content	Evaluation
1. The student participants will be able to (in their interaction with each other and patient being interviewed) describe asthma, its definition, pathophysiological aspects, differential diagnosis, risk factors, anatomical issues, S&S, disease presentation, and treatment, including treatment risks. This content will be applied in the clinical presentation of a case study.	The student participants will be able to identify the following: 1. Risk factors for asthma, including age, environmental risk, allergens, VOG, pollution 2. Presenting S&S, including use of accessory muscles, DOE, circumoral and peripheral cyanosis, panic 3. Treatment including bronchodilators, steroids, respiratory treatments at home 4. Patient teaching including exercise, use of meds, complications of meds 5. Complications: including status asthmaticus, respiratory decompensation	—Causative agents and risk factors for asthma —Pathophysiology of asthma —Anticipated ABG changes —Clinical presentation from mild to severe presentation —Anticipated treatment —Complications	Students who met outcomes: Student 1:_____ Student 2:_____ Student 3:_____ Student 4:_____ Student 5:_____ Student 6:_____

(continued)

Objectives	Outcomes	Course Content	Evaluation
2. In the course of clinical rounds, students will demonstrate IPR and team skills.			Student 1:_____ Student 2:_____ Student 3:_____ Student 4:_____ Student 5:_____ Student 6:_____
3. In the course of clinical rounds, students will demonstrate appropriate, role-specific professional skills.			Student 1:_____ Student 2:_____ Student 3:_____ Student 4:_____ Student 5:_____ Student 6:_____
4. The student leader will be able to guide the student group through the content specific to the issue under discussion and the issues related to clinical and nursing care.			If a student led, comments on performance:
5. The student providing the "patient" case study will be able to provide a case illustration of the issues under discussion during clinical rounds.		—Presentation of a case study by a student	If a student was the patient, comments:

APPENDIX 20

Grading Rubric for Clinical Rounds Learning Acitvity 15: Osteoporosis

Date: _____   Group: _____

Student 1: _____   Student 2: _____   Student 3: _____

Student 4: _____   Student 5: _____   Student 6: _____

Student leader, if utilized: _____   Student in patient role, if utilized: _____

Objectives	Outcomes	Course Content	Evaluation
1. The student participants will be able to (in their interaction with each other and patient being interviewed) describe the following for osteoporosis: —S&S —Care issues —Treatment	The student participants will be able to identify the following: —Risk factors —Diagnosis, treatment, and patient teaching for behavior modification and management of risk factors The student group will be able to respond to questions about content and care planning by the clinical rounds leader.	—Risk factors: related to fractures and early mortality, estrogen deficiency, European and Asian ancestry are at increased risk, small stature, tobacco, malnutrition —Dx: bone mineral density studies, radiology, DXA study —Tx: lifestyle changes, vitamin D, calcium in some populations, bisphosphonates —Teaching: diet, exercise (weight bearing) and fall prevention: NOT necessarily advisable to take calcium and vitamin D	Students who met outcomes: Student 1:_____ Student 2:_____ Student 3:_____ Student 4:_____ Student 5:_____ Student 6:_____

(continued)

Objectives	Outcomes	Course Content	Evaluation
2. Students will in the course of clinical rounds demonstrate IPR and team skills.			Student 1:_____ Student 2:_____ Student 3:_____ Student 4:_____ Student 5:_____ Student 6:_____
3. In the course of clinical rounds, students will demonstrate appropriate, role-specific professional skills.			Student 1:_____ Student 2:_____ Student 3:_____ Student 4:_____ Student 5:_____ Student 6:_____
4. The student leader will be able to guide the student group through the content specific to the issue under discussion and the issues related to clinical and nursing care.			If a student led, comments on performance:
5. The student providing the "patient" case study will be able to provide a case illustration of the issues under discussion during clinical rounds.		—Presentation of a case study by a student	If a student was the patient, comments:

APPENDIX 21

Grading Rubric for Clinical Rounds Learning Activity 16: Hyponatremia

Date: _____   Group: _____

Student 1: _____   Student 2: _____   Student 3: _____

Student 4: _____   Student 5: _____   Student 6: _____

Student leader, if utilized: _____   Student in patient role, if utilized: _____

Objective	Outcomes	Course Content	Students
1. The student participants will be able to (in their interaction with each other and patient being interviewed) describe hyponatremia. This content will be applied in the clinical presentation of a case study.	The student participants will be able to identify the following: risk factors (including lifestyle), underlying pathophysiology, signs and symptoms, complications, treatment, and typical presentation The student group will be able to respond to questions about content and care planning by the clinical rounds leader.	Review of definition of hyponatremia: —Risk factors (including lifestyle) —Pathophysiology —S&S and complications (across all systems) including neuro, CV, and M/S —Treatment —Presentation of a case study by a student	Students who met outcomes: Student 1:_____ Student 2:_____ Student 3:_____ Student 4:_____ Student 5:_____ Student 6:_____
2. In the course of clinical rounds, students will demonstrate IPR and team skills.			Student 1:_____ Student 2:_____ Student 3:_____ Student 4:_____ Student 5:_____ Student 6:_____

(continued)

Objective	Outcomes	Course Content	Students
3. In the course of clinical rounds, students will demonstrate appropriate, role-specific professional skills.			Student 1:_____ Student 2:_____ Student 3:_____ Student 4:_____ Student 5:_____ Student 6:_____
4. The student leader will be able to guide the student group through the content specific to the issue under discussion and the issues related to clinical and nursing care.	The student leader will provide the group questions that relate to the above content and to supplement the group discussion with relevant additional content.		If a student led, comments on performance:
5. The student providing the "patient" case study will be able to provide a case illustration of the issues under discussion during clinical rounds.	The patient will provide meaningful, content-specific examples of the issues being discussed in clinical rounds.		If a student was the patient, comments:

APPENDIX 22

Grading Rubric for Clinical Rounds Learning Activity 17: Pituitary Function and Pathology

Date: _____   Group: _____

Student 1: _____   Student 2: _____   Student 3: _____

Student 4: _____   Student 5: _____   Student 6: _____

Student leader, if utilized: _____   Student in patient role, if utilized: _____

Objective	Outcomes	Course Content	Evaluation
1. The student participants will be able to (in their interaction with each other and patient being interviewed) describe the structure, function, and pathology associated with the pituitary gland.	The student participants will be able to identify the following: —Role of the pituitary gland —Role of releasing factors and feedback cycles in hormonal regulation —Causes of hyper/hypothyroidism —S/S of hyper/hypothyroidism —Important factors to identify in a patient presenting with pituitary disease —Treatment of a patient presenting with pituitary disease	Primary function of the pituitary gland: —"Master gland" —Controls function of endocrine organs —Maintains homeostasis, controls metabolism and growth —Excretes releasing factors that stimulate the activity of ACTH, GH, LH, TH, FSH —Regulation of hormones via feedback cycles and releasing factors Describe HPA axis Causes and manifestations of hyper/hypopituitarism	Students who met outcomes: Student 1:_____ Student 2:_____ Student 3:_____ Student 4:_____ Student 5:_____ If a student led, comments on performance: If a student was the patient, comments:

(continued)

Objective	Outcomes	Course Content	Evaluation
2. In the course of clinical rounds, students will demonstrate IPR and team skills.			Student 1:_____ Student 2:_____ Student 3:_____ Student 4:_____ Student 5:_____ Student 6:_____
3. In the course of clinical rounds, students will demonstrate appropriate, role-specific professional skills.			Student 1:_____ Student 2:_____ Student 3:_____ Student 4:_____ Student 5:_____ Student 6:_____
4. The student providing the "patient" case study will be able to provide a case illustration of the issues under discussion during clinical rounds.		The patient will provide meaningful, content-specific examples of the issues being discussed in clinical rounds.	If a student was the patient, comments:

APPENDIX 23

Grading Rubric for Clinical Rounds Learning Activity 18: Peripheral Vascular Disease

Date: _____   Group: _____

Student 1: _____   Student 2: _____   Student 3: _____

Student 4: _____   Student 5: _____   Student 6: _____

Student leader, if utilized: _____   Student in patient role, if utilized: _____

Objectives	Outcomes	Course Content	Evaluation
1. The student participants will be able to (in their interaction with each other and patient being interviewed) describe peripheral vascular disease, its definition, pathophysiological aspects, differentiation of emboli and thrombus, risk factors, anatomical issues, S&S, disease presentation, and treatment, including treatment risks. This content will be applied in the clinical presentation of a case study.	The student participants will be able to identify the following: (See course content definition of PVD) The student group will be able to respond to questions about content and care planning by the clinical rounds leader.	Review of definition of PVD: —Risk factors (including lifestyle) —Pathophysiology —Difference between emboli and thrombus —S&S (including color, sensation, blanching, pulse changes) —Treatment including anticoagulants and their complications —Presentation of a case study by a student	Students who met outcomes: Student 1:_____ Student 2:_____ Student 3:_____ Student 4:_____ Student 5:_____ Student 6:_____

(continued)

Objectives	Outcomes	Course Content	Evaluation
2. In the course of clinical rounds, students will demonstrate IPR and team skills.			Student 1:_____ Student 2:_____ Student 3:_____ Student 4:_____ Student 5:_____ Student 6:_____
3. In the course of clinical rounds, students will demonstrate appropriate, role-specific professional skills.			Student 1:_____ Student 2:_____ Student 3:_____ Student 4:_____ Student 5:_____ Student 6:_____
4. The student leader will be able to guide the student group through the content specific to the issue under discussion and the issues related to clinical and nursing care.			If a student led, comments on performance:
5. The student providing the "patient" case study will be able to provide a case illustration of the issues under discussion during clinical rounds.			If a student was the patient, comments:

APPENDIX 24

Grading Rubric for Clinical Rounds Learning Activity 19: Pneumonia

Date: _____   Group: _____

Student 1: _____   Student 2: _____   Student 3: _____

Student 4: _____   Student 5: _____   Student 6: _____

Student leader, if utilized: _____   Student in patient role, if utilized: _____

Objective	Outcomes	Course Content	Evaluation
1. During the patient interview, the patient (presenting the case study) or the nurse (assessing and diagnosing the patient) will identify historical, lifestyle risk factors and clinical signs of bacterial pneumonia.	The student participants will be able to identify the following: (Note course content for causative factors and clinical presentation) The student group will be able to respond to questions about content and care planning by the clinical rounds leader.	Causative factors considered: —Immunosuppression, malnutrition, environmental exposure —SOB, dyspnea on exertion, decreased breath sounds, cyanosis, tachycardia, hyper then hypotension, mental status changes	Students who met outcomes: Student 1:_____ Student 2:_____ Student 3:_____ Student 4:_____ Student 5:_____
2. Pertinent labs and diagnostic tests will be reviewed (Dialogue and SOAP).		Decreased Po_2, increased CO_2, increased WBC, infiltrates on CXR	If a student led, comments on performance:

(continued)

Objective	Outcomes	Course Content	Evaluation
3. A differential diagnosis will be established and the diagnosis for the patient substantiated (SOAP).		—Status asthmaticus, COPD, viral pneumonia, bronchitis	If a student was the patient, comments:
4. Treatment plan will be reviewed with the patient (dialogue).		—Rehydration —Antibiotics —Nutrition —Hospitalization/ EKG monitoring if patient does not stabilize —Observation for sepsis and multisystem complications	
5. Education plan elucidated (SOAP).		—Prevention, early S&S	
6. Students will in the course of clinical rounds demonstrate IPR and team skills.			Student 1:_____ Student 2:_____ Student 3:_____ Student 4:_____ Student 5:_____ Student 6:_____
7. In the course of clinical rounds, students will demonstrate appropriate, role-specific professional skills.			Student 1:_____ Student 2:_____ Student 3:_____ Student 4:_____ Student 5:_____ Student 6:_____

(continued)

Objective	Outcomes	Course Content	Evaluation
8. The student leader will be able to guide the student group through the content specific to the issue under discussion and the issues related to clinical and nursing care.			If a student led, comments on performance:
9. The student providing the "patient" case study will be able to provide a case illustration of the issues under discussion during clinical rounds.		—Presentation of a case study by a student	If a student was the patient, comments:

APPENDIX 25

Clinical Rounds: Template for Planning a Pathology-Focused Learning Activity

Date: _____   Group: _____

Student 1: _____   Student 2: _____   Student 3: _____

Student 4: _____   Student 5: _____   Student 6: _____

Student leader, if utilized: _____   Student in patient role, if utilized: _____

Objectives	Outcomes	Course Content	Evaluation
1. The student participants will be able to (in their interaction with the each other and patient being interviewed) describe _____, its definition, pathophysiological aspects, differential diagnosis, risk factors, anatomical issues, S&S, disease presentation, and treatment, including treatment risks. This content will be applied in the clinical presentation of a case study.	The student group will be able to respond to questions about content and care planning by the clinical rounds leader, based upon specific course content related to the specific pathology.		Students who met outcomes: Student 1:_____ Student 2:_____ Student 3:_____ Student 4:_____ Student 5:_____
2. The student leader will be able to guide the student group through the content specific to the issue under discussion and the issues related to clinical and nursing care.			If a student led, comments on performance:

(continued)

Objectives	Outcomes	Course Content	Evaluation
3. The student providing the "patient" case study will be able to provide a case illustration of the issues under discussion during clinical rounds.		—Presentation of a case study by a student	If a student was the patient, comments:

APPENDIX 26

Student Introduction to Second Life®

What Is Second Life®?

Second Life® is a virtual world. It is a world of "islands" where you can find cities, beaches, forests, universities, and even places from the future and past! The graphics for Second Life® are three-dimensional and realistic—you will hear birds singing and see the wind blowing through trees!

In Second Life®, people do the same things they do in "First Life" (our regular usual lives!). There are places to go (rainforests, planets from the future, places from the past, shopping areas, art galleries, music venues, gardens, universities) and many things to do (windsurfing, hot air ballooning, looking into microscopes, exploring a giant chromosome). There are people to interact with from all over the world. (You will see and hear people talking many languages.) Second Life® is a great place to learn—want to tour a "Virtual Stomach" or walk through a "chromosome forest"?

Second Life® is also a place where people can meet for conversations, interactions, and many different of kinds of learning!

How Do I Go to Second Life®?

To enter Second Life®, you need to make your Second Life® body, which is called an "avatar." This is the body that you will walk, run, dance, and fly with in Second Life® and the "person" who will interact with others in Second Life®.

To begin, you will need to Google "Second Life®" or just go to Secondlife .com. The main website for Second Life® will tell you how to begin. This will involve downloading the (free) Second Life® software, setting up an account, making a Second Life® name for yourself, and creating your avatar. (Note: please use your real first name so identifying classmates will be easier!). If you have difficulty with any of the orientation activities, notify your instructor.

Is Second Life® a Game?

No, Second Life® is not a game, although you can play all sorts of games there if you want to. Second Life® is a world, with the same activities that take place in "First World," like learning, which brings us to . . .

Why Is Second Life® a Part of This Course?

One of the most powerful developments in nursing education in the last few years is called "Simulation Lab." In simulation, you get to practice things that you will be doing in the real world of your clinical practice. Simulation is a great way of learning. In this course, we will be using Second Life® as a simulation to put ethics into practice in a variety of ways. Imagine participating in "Virtual clinical rounds" where we go to a virtual hospital and do clinical rounds on a patient together to discuss ethical issues. Or, we may choose to meet in a classroom (lots of universities have "Virtual Campuses" in Second Life®) or maybe we will meet around a campfire on the beach for a discussion group!

Why Haven't I Heard of Second Life® in School Before?

Second Life® is not new—it has been around for a while—but educators are just beginning to catch on to the potential it has for effective and interesting learning. Lots of universities have Second Life® campuses. Second Life® is just beginning to be used in nursing education, so we will be learning together about how best to use it!

Will It Take a Long Time to Learn How to Use Second Life®?

This varies a lot in terms of how tech-savvy you are and how interested you are in Second Life ®. For this course, you will be using only very basic Second Life® skills. You will NOT be shopping, building a house, throwing a party, or even changing clothing (although of course you could do those things on your own time if you like). Some startup learning will be involved, and it will take a while to get up to speed. Lots of help will be available. For all of this course, you will be considered a "newbie" (this is Second Life® language for someone who has spent less than 30 hours in Second Life®), which means only very basic things will be required of you.

Is There Special "Lingo" That Goes Along with Second Life®?

Well, you have heard some already—yes, and there is a lot of Second Life®–specific language. For the purposes of this course, please be familiar with the terms on the attached Second Life® terminology page.

Are There Special "Customs" in Second Life®?

Second Life® has some specific behavioral expectations that will be included in your orientation to Second Life®. In general, common sense applies—don't bother other people!

Bad Behavior

There is little "policing" in Second Life®, and some people's idea of fun is to set fire to others' projects. If you are bumped/followed/harassed/annoyed by another person in Second Life®, the best thing to do is LEAVE. Either teleport somewhere else or sign off Second Life®. It is a good idea to report the annoyance. People are suspended from Second Life® activity if they bother others.

Being new, you will probably stumble around, make mistakes, and inadvertently annoy other people. All you have to say is "newbie"—this tells others you are just learning!

Privacy

Do NOT use your real last name when naming your avatar. You should not give out private information to anyone in Second Life®. It is considered VERY RUDE to ask it of others in Second Life®.

Communicating in Second Life®

There are lots of ways to communicate in Second Life®, including using a real voice. The easiest way, and the only way that we will use for this course, is typing your messages, which appear on the Second Life® screen of anyone near you. This is the only form of communication that will be used for the course.

Does Second Life® Cost Anything?

Second Life® software is free. "Inworld" (which means "in Second Life®"), there is a whole Second Life® economy, based on currency called Linden™

dollars. It is possible to go shopping, buy property, build houses, etc. Some people have "jobs" in Second Life® that they use to earn a Linden™ dollars! THIS COURSE WILL NOT REQUIRE ANY MONETARY ACTIVITIES.

What If I Have Trouble Learning Second Life®?

The course instructor will do orientation for the class and will be offering periodic extra help sessions and one-on-one sessions if needed. If you get lost or confused, don't worry—help is available! "Inworld" there is lots of help available as well, and remember, this is a populated world, so don't hesitate to ask for help of the others.

What If I Am Already Familiar with Second Life® and/or Have a Second Life® Avatar?

If you are already "inworld" and already have an avatar there, let your instructor know in case a name change for your avatar is needed.

What If My Computer Does Not Meet Specifications for the Second Life® Software?

The computers in your school or library may have Second Life® installed. You can do Second Life® activities there if it is not possible to download the Second Life® viewer on your home computer.

What about Mature Content?

In some areas of Second Life®, there are locations and activities related to mature content. This includes content of a sexual/violent/rude nature. These are NOT included in course activities; it is the responsibility of the student to avoid mature content areas/activities. If at any point you are uncomfortable with the environment or behavior of another avatar, just sign out of Second Life®, and make sure you discuss the problem with your instructor.

Before You Begin

Before starting out, please review the following expectations for Second Life® in this course:

1. Avatar Name: As you set up your account, you will be asked to make a name for your avatar. For the purposes of this course, you MUST use your "real" (First Life) name. You can use any second name you like.

2. Appearance: Please keep your appearance "professional," meaning no nudity, overexposed skin, weird hats, wings, tails, or bizarre stuff. Basically, nothing you wouldn't wear to class. If you want to, you can explore changing clothing from that which you are "born" in (avatars that are being created are "being born"), but that should NOT be included in the time you spend on the class.

3. Second Life® Language: There are some basic Second Life® terms that will be used both in class and in Second Life®. Please review them before you begin.

4. "Talking" in Second Life®: Although it is possible to put on headphones with a microphone and talk live in Second Life®, for the purpose of this course, you will be typing your talking—that way, a copy of the discussion can be kept. In the lower left-hand part of the screen is a chat option that should be used for all course communication.

Use of Second Life® in this course is relatively new, so you will be asked to evaluate how useful it has been. Please include your feedback in all course and instructor evaluations related to the course.

READY TO BEGIN? Check out "Second Life® Language" then GO TO Secondlife.com and click on "Get Started." If at any point you need help, e-mail your instructor. If you are nervous about the whole idea, e-mail your instructor. He or she will be happy to walk you through it.

Second Life® "Language"

Term Definition/Example of Usage

Second Life®	This refers to the registered virtual world of Second Life®.
"First Life"	This refers to the world outside of Second Life®—that is to say, your regular life! As in, "Nice talking to you but I have to go back to first life!"
"Inworld"	This refers to what goes on in Second Life®, or being in Second Life®, as in "See you inworld." That means, "See you in Second Life®!"
Avatar	Your Second Life® body/persona, complete with a body, a name, and clothing.
Newbie	A newbie is someone who is new to Second Life®. By definition, this is someone who has spent less than 30 hours in

	Second Life®. Newbies tend to look funny and act funny (falling off walls, getting stuck in trees, etc.). If you do something weird when someone else is around (bump into them, etc.), all you have to "say" is "newbie." This is shorthand for, "Cut me a little slack, I don't know how to walk yet!"
Griefing	Griefing is "inappropriate behavior" in Second Life®. If another person bothers you in Second Life®, he or she is "griefing" you. Griefing should be reported and can result in others being exiled from Second Life®.
Born	An avatar is "born" the day the avatar is created.
Postcard	A "Postcard" is a way to take a picture of where you are in Second Life® and send it by e-mail. We will be using postcards as a way to validate your Second Life® activities. For instructions on how to send a postcard, see "Second Life® 'How to' Tips."
Lag	Lag is the pause that happens while the graphics for Second Life® form. When you teleport to a new place, it takes a minute or so for the world to "form" around you. Depending on your computer and some other factors, lag can be minimal or more severe.

Second Life® "How to" Tips

Once you have a Second Life® account and a body and have begun some orientation to Second Life® (Orientation Island and other areas for new people in Second Life®), you might benefit from the following tips:

How to Search for a Particular Location

1. Search Options:

   a. **General Searching:** On the bottom of your Second Life® screen, click on SEARCH. On the top of the search menu, you can select what you want to search for: A place? A person? For example, if you are interested in looking at treehouses, type it in and click SEARCH. All Second Life® locations that have treehouses will appear. This is the easiest way to search, but it doesn't include everything.

   A list of search results will show up. Click on one and a popup description of the area will appear. If you want to go to that area, click on "teleport."

b. **The Second Life® Map:** Second Life® has large maps that you can also use to search. Click on MAPS. This will bring up a large map screen of Second Life®. Along the right-hand side of that screen, you will see a "search" option. In that area, type a word that relates to what you are looking for. It might be a specific place, like "Reflection Island" or "Info Island." Or, it could be someplace you would like to explore, for example, "rainforest" or "treehouses." In the area below, a list of places related to that search word will appear. Click on the one that interests you! You can also type in specific coordinates that you want to teleport to; locations used for meetings, etc., in this course will use specific coordinates.

c. **Coordinates:** On the same right-hand side of the map screen is a place where you can indicate the map coordinates of a known location. For example, if a group meeting is set for coordinates 119-147-22, you can type in those coordinates. You have to include the island that the location is on.

How to "Speak"

On the lower left-hand part of your screen, you will see an option called COMMUNICATE. Click on that and select "Local Chat." Type in what you would like to say. Anyone around you in Second Life® will see your chatting appear on their screen and have the option of replying. (Although we will not use it for this course, automatic translation software is available in Second Life® that enables you to communicate with people speaking other languages.)

How to Send a Postcard

We will be using postcards a lot. On the lower left of the screen, select "Snapshot." Use the screen to send the snapshot in an e-mail. In several of your early assignments, you will need to send a snapshot to the course coordinator or your instructor.

How to Report "Griefing"

If anyone bothers you, write down his or her name. Also note your location (this is always along the top of the screen) and the time of day. Next, right click to bring up your circle of options. Keep clicking on "more" until you come to "Report." Click on this to file a griefing report. This is also useful if something bizarre happens around you (suddenly everyone is in cages, etc.).

APPENDIX 27

Student Checklist: Orientation to Second Life®

_____ Download Second Life® software

_____ Sign up for basic, free Second Life® membership

_____ Create an avatar name (real first name only for students, "Student Robert")

_____ Create an avatar (professionally appropriate in appearance, must be human)

_____ Proficiency in walking, teleporting, sitting

_____ Proficiency in use of chat box for communication

_____ Copying of chat dialogue into a Word file

_____Confirmed access to wired Internet

Orientation completed on _____ (Date) Student signature: _____

Second Life® avatar name: _____

Please return this form, signed, to your course instructor.

APPENDIX 28

Instructor Checklist: Orientation to Second Life®

Navigation Skills

Walking, running, flying, teleporting _____

Teleporting between regions and within regions _____

Jumping and aerial maneuvering to get out of water, off cliffs, etc. _____

Student rescue skills: talking students through unstuck, out of water, etc. _____

Maneuvering: around obstacles, through complex building structures _____

Student rescue skills: how to send an offer to teleport to the instructor's location _____

Communication

Chat box: facile use of chat box, copying and saving dialogue, dealing with lag _____

IM communication for private messages to students _____

Region Skills

Able to search Second Life® for regions appropriate for learning activities _____

Able to identify region qualities that would support learning _____

Able to identify mature content in an environment inappropriate for a learning activity _____

Able to change regional lighting to make it appropriate for a learning activity _____

Able to assist students with managing lag if it occurs _____

Avatar Maintenance

Able to open new accounts to create multiple avatars _____

Able to modify personal avatar to support professionalism and leader maturity _____

Able to modify patient avatars' appearance to manifest physical symptoms of disease _____

Able to manage multiple avatars on one computer screen _____

Able to manage two roles during a learning activity (patient and group leader) _____

Able to change clothing for an avatar to support a learning activity _____

Able to change an avatar's age _____

Privacy Maintenance

Able to identify regions that maintain maximal privacy _____

Able to support students' privacy and reinforce limits on self-disclosure if needed _____

Griefing

Able to report griefing when necessary _____

Able to reinforce importance of reporting griefing during orientation _____

APPENDIX 29

Emotional Intelligence Learning Activity 20: EI Ability Observed in Public Interactions

Background: This course has identified three main models of emotional intelligence: the Ability Model, the Personality Model, and the Mixed Model. For the purposes of this assignment, each student will choose one of these models for use in the assignment. Using the model, students will observe Second Life® residents' behavior in some public Second Life® region and evaluate their interactions in terms of EI attributes according to that model.

Assignment Goal: The purpose of this assignment is for each student to identify EI attributes in Second Life® residents' interactions observed in a public region in Second Life®.

Assignment Steps:

1. Identify a region or location in Second Life® where there is a lot of interaction between avatars.

2. Observe interactions in this region for 30 minutes and assess the interactions in terms of EI attributes.

3. Include in the observations examples of specific EI attributes or abilities, as well as examples of interactions that could have been improved by use of an EI attribute or ability.

4. After the observation, do an evaluation of use of the EI model. Which aspects of the model were illustrated (in its presence or absence in the interaction)? Which elements were not? Was this model useful in observing interactions or not?

Submission Format: This assignment should be submitted in a Word document attached to an e-mail to the instructor.

Grading matrix: This is a simple introductory assignment that will be graded on an A-B-C-D-F basis according to the following grading rubric:

Grading Rubric

Grading Criteria	Total Points Possible	Points Achieved	Comments
1. List of EI attributes observed	30		
2. List of EI attributes not observed or evident in interactions	30		
3. Summary evaluation (Was the model useful?)	30		
4. Assignment is submitted on time (8 a.m. Friday; all or nothing points)	5		
5. Assignment is submitted in the required format (all or nothing points)	5		
Total points	100		

APPENDIX 30

Emotional Intelligence Learning
Activity 21: Quest 1

These are the directions for an emotional intelligence teamwork learning activity in Second Life® called "Quest 1."

Quest 1 takes place at the Second Life® location called "Irreplaceable."

Do NOT check out this location before your group quest!

The Quest 1 assignment has two parts:

1. First you will spend 30 to 60 minutes (no longer, please) together at the Second Life® location "Irresistible," attempting to complete Quest 1.

2. After the quest, send your group report and the dialogue to the instructor RIGHT AWAY.

3. AFTER RECIEVING THE DIALOGUE AND GROUP REPORT, the instructor will send the group the data analysis sheet to use to complete a quantitative analysis of Quest 1. Each student will complete the analysis and report on it for the paper that is due later in the course.

Notes for Completing Quest 1:

Quest 1 is a teamwork analysis project, so it has both outcome objectives (locate the objects on the list and locate the pirate treasure) and teamwork objectives (how the group performs on their objectives for team performance, as well as the objectives the instructor will have you include in the paper).

Quest 1 will require some flying, the ability to sit on things, and some picture taking! THESE you might want to practice before the group meets. To FLY, click on the WALK/FLY/RUN part of the icon bar at the bottom of the Second Life® screen: click on the icon that looks like flying. TO SIT, right click on the item you want to sit on and select "sit" from the drop-down menu. TO SEND A POSTCARD, on the far left of the Second Life® screen, click on the bottom icon that looks like a camera; it will walk you through the steps. You will be sending the instructor several postcards as part of completing the quest. If you need help on any of this, let the instructor know. For the postcard, use the instructor's e-mail or one provided.

Disclaimer: This site is identified as an ADULT site. The instructor can't figure out why, so if you stumble on something ADULT, steer clear . . . the quest *doesn't* involve sex, drugs, or violence!

Steps for Quest 1:

1. Print out this page so you can refer to it as the quest progresses.

2. Make a time for the group to meet in "Irreplaceable."

3. Once you are in the landing area, have a brief group meeting. The group needs to FIRST identify FIVE things you will be able to look back on in the dialogue to measure the teamwork effectiveness.

4. Once you have identified the five things, the quest can begin. (It might be a good idea for the group to review the RULES before beginning.) Violation of the rules results in points deductions!

Rules:
- At all times, the group has to have an identified leader. The leader role changes every 10 minutes.

- The group must stay together: the rough equivalent of 50 feet (if you can't see what is being said in the chat dialogue, you are too far away).

- (This isn't a rule but a suggestion: a timekeeper might be a good idea!)

Quest 1 Goals:

1. Locate the pirate treasure and send a postcard to the instructor with the whole group around the treasure.

   HINT: The treasure is not where you think it would be, and if it is found, it most likely will be found FAILING at one of the other quest objectives.

2. Locate the following items/perform the following/answer the following questions (these will be included in the report to your instructor:

- Pay your respects at the grave of Nannie Connie . . . who does she hang out with these days?

- Identify the following animals (include in your report where you found them): horse, peacock, deer.

- What does the group think the most important vow is?

- As a group, sit around a fireplace or campfire and send the instructor a postcard of the group.

- What is the largest star on the Second Life®?

- Name one item inside the treehouse.

- Take a picture of one of the group members sitting on the raft at the vortex.

- If you are steering the pirate ship, what do you see?

- Take a postcard picture of the group in the castle hot tub and send it to the instructor.

WHEN THE QUEST IS COMPLETED (when you have completed the quest or when time runs out):

1. Identify one person to send the dialogue and the group's answers to the Quest Questions to the instructor.

2. Once the instructor has gotten the dialogue and report, she will send the group the data analysis questions and directions for the paper that is due.

Any questions? Drop the instructor a note!

APPENDIX 31

Quest 1 Data Analysis Paper: Quantitative Measures Assignment

Quest Purpose: The purpose of this exploratory quantitative study is to describe the elements of team effectiveness for the Quest 1 team. Specific research questions include the following:

1. Is there evidence of effective leadership for the team in Quest 1?

2. Is effective team communication illustrated in the Quest 1 team?

3. Was the team able to meet performance objectives?

A data analysis grid will be utilized to gather the data from the Quest 1 dialogue transcript that will be used to answer these three questions.

Steps for the Assignment:

FIRST: On the Quest 1 assignment dialogue, de-identify the names of all the participants in the quest. To do this, use "FIND" in Word, and one at a time put in one of the team member's name. Then add "REPLACE," and put in a number that identifies that person. Once you do this, for example, "HUHJohn" gets replaced with "Team Member 3."

Print out the dialogue with the names changed to code names/numbers.

SECOND: Use the data analysis grid to collect data from the dialogue transcript.

THIRD: Write a two-page paper to summarize BRIEFLY the findings of the data analysis.

Data Analysis and Evaluation Chart

Criterion 1: Leadership	Rationale	Benchmark	Data from Dialogue
1. Leadership changes every 10 minutes per rules	Rules of the quest	One change per 10 minutes of the quest:	_____ minutes _____ leader changes
2. At least four people from the group had a period of leadership	In effective teams, leadership, both informal and formal, is SHARED in the group, not dominated by one or a few people	4	_____ Number of different leaders
3. The group followed the leader's directions	For leadership to be effective, team members have to be willing to follow!	The group follows at least 75 percent of the directions they received from the leaders on the quest	_____ Total number of leader directions for the _____ Number of directions the group followed
4. At least once, the group disagrees with the leader	For leadership to be effective, the leader has to be willing to change his or her mind on the basis of feedback from the group	At least once on the quest, a group member disagreed with the leader At least once, the leader changed his or her mind on the basis of group input	_____ Total number of times someone disagreed with the leader _____ Total number of times the leader changed his or her mind
5. At least once, the leader affirmed group performance	Affirmation of positive team performance from the leader enhances team effectiveness and has a positive effect on motivation of team members	At least once, one of the leaders affirmed positive team performance	_____ Total number of times a leader affirmed the team
6. At least once, a leader gave the team feedback on how to improve	Constructive team feedback enhances performance and both individual and group learning	At least once, one of the leaders offered constructive feedback	_____ Total number of times a leader offered constructive feedback
LEADERSHIP SUBSCORE		90 percent	

(continued)

Criterion 2: Communication	Rationale	Benchmark	Data from Dialogue
1. All team members contribute regularly to the performance of the group	Participation of all group members means each is bringing his or her gifts to the group task and no member is "dead weight"	Of the total number of times someone spoke for the whole duration of the quest, each team member represents at least 10 percent of the number of dialogue entries	_____ Total number of dialogue entries Percentage for each group member: 1. _____ 2. _____ 3. _____ 4. _____ 5. _____ 6. _____
2. Team members give each other feedback responses on each other's input: affirmation, presenting alternative views, etc.	Team effectiveness improves when team members respond to each other! The "give-and-take" between team members about the task at hand improves chances of meeting the team goals creatively and effectively.	There are at least 10 examples throughout the dialogue of team members responding to each other's ideas	___ Total number of dialogue entries that exhibit team members responding to each other
Criterion 3: Meeting Team Goals			
1. The team is able to identify measurable criteria for evaluating their quest performance	A team that is able to set measures of their effectiveness has a greater chance of measurable success	The team will be able to identify five MEASURABLE goals (including HOW they will be measured) that are specific to team performance	Number of goals identified:_____ Number of goals that were measurable (means of measurement identified)_____ Number of these goals that relate to team performance:____

(continued)

2. The team is able to achieve the identified goals for the quest	Team performance is largely measured by fulfillment of identified goals and outcomes	The team met the assignment objectives: ___4 Objects located ___4 Questions answered ___3 Postcards	1. The pirate treasure was located:_____ 2. Number of postcards sent to instructor:_____ 3. Number of items located correctly:_____ 4. Number of questions answered correctly____
3. The team is able to meet the objectives it set for itself		1. Efficiency (time between tasks) 2. Number of negative comments? 3. Chat participation? 4. Conversation effectiveness? 5. Completed tasks?	

SUMMARIZE the findings of the Quest 1 data collection in a two-page paper. No sources are required for this paper, but use correct APA structure (headings, pagination). NO title page is required. The following structure is recommended:

1. Introduction to team effectiveness

2. Purpose statement and research questions

3. Description of study procedures

4. Findings: What were the answers to the research questions?

APPENDIX 32

Emotional Intelligence Learning Activity 22: Quest 2 EI Attributes

Quest 2 takes place at the Second Life® location called "Irreplaceable."
Do NOT check out this location before your group quest!

The Quest 2 assignment has two parts:

1. First you will spend 30 to 60 minutes (no longer, please) together at the Second Life® location "Irresistible," attempting to complete the quest.

2. After the quest, send your group report and the dialogue to the instructor RIGHT AWAY.

3. AFTER RECIEVING THE DIALOGUE AND GROUP REPORT, the instructor will send the group the data analysis sheet to use to complete a quantitative analysis of the quest. Each student will complete the analysis and report on it for the paper that is due later in the course.

Notes for Completing the Quest:

Quest 2 is a teamwork analysis project, so it has both outcome objectives (locate the objects on the list and the pirate treasure, answer the questions) and emotional intelligence objectives. Once you complete the quest, the instructor will send you the analysis grid that will help you collect data for your paper.

Remember, for postcards, send your postcard to the instructor.

Disclaimer: This site is identified as an ADULT site. The instructor can't figure out why, so if you stumble on something ADULT, steer clear . . . the quest *doesn't* involve sex, drugs, or violence!

To open doors, or objects (like treasure chests), right click on the object.

Steps for Quest 2:

1. Print out this page so you can refer to it as the quest progresses.

2. Make a time for the group to meet in "Irreplaceable."

3. Once you are in the landing area, have a brief group meeting. During this time, review the rules and goals for the quest.

Rules:

1. The group must stay together: the rough equivalent of 50 feet (if you can't see what is being said in the chat dialogue, you are too far away).

2. The quest can take ONLY 60 minutes!

Emotional Intelligence Goals (You Might Want to Think about These before You Start)

The EI goal is for each student to demonstrate as many EI attributes as possible sometime during the quest. EACH student will keep a tally of when each student illustrates an EI attribute. On the log, the TIME should be logged onto the EI attributes chart when the student illustrated it. (Keep track of yourself, also.) The EI attributes chart and operational definitions are found in Appendix 33.

Quest Goals:

1. Locate the pirate treasure and send a postcard to the instructor with the whole group around the treasure.

   HINT: There is a second pirate ship: you might find it accidently while you are pursuing another goal.

2. Locate the following items/perform the following/answer the following questions:

- Is there debris from when Atlantis sunk? How many columns remain below?

- What does the group think the most important vow is?

- As a group, sit around the castle fireplace. Send the instructor a postcard of the group there.

- What creature guards the castle, and what is it being fed?

- Who stands guard on the castle tower?

- What is the miller's hobby?

- Send a postcard of the group from the miller's living room.

- Where is the octopus?

- Take a picture of one of the group members in a hammock.

WHEN THE QUEST IS COMPLETED (when you have completed the quest, or when time runs out):

1. Identify one person to send the dialogue to the instructor.

2. Once the instructor has gotten the dialogue and report, she will send the group the data analysis questions and directions for the paper that is due.

Any questions? Drop the instructor a note!

APPENDIX 33

Emotional Intelligence Attributes Chart and Operational Definitions

Students:	1	2	3	4	5	6
Self-regard						
Emotional self-awareness						
Assertiveness						
Independence						
Self-actualization						
Empathy						
Social responsibility						
Interpersonal relationships						
Reality testing						
Flexibility						
Problem solving						
Stress tolerance						

(continued)

Students:	1	2	3	4	5	6
Impulse control						
Optimism						
Happiness						

Operational Definitions for Emotional Intelligence (Personality Model)

Attribute	Operational Definition
Self-regard	Respect for and acceptance of one's self.
Emotional self-awareness	Recognition of one's feelings and what caused them.
Assertiveness	Expression and defense of feelings, beliefs, thoughts, and rights in a nondestructive way.
Independence	Self-direction and self-control, emotional independence.
Self-actualization	Realization of potential capabilities.
Empathy	Awareness of, understanding, and appreciation of the feelings of others.
Social responsibility	Cooperation, constructive, and contributing membership in a social group.
Interpersonal relationships	Making and maintaining positive relationships and a positive work environment.
Reality testing	Assessment of differences between what is being experienced and what is objectively happening.
Flexibility	Adjustment to a changing situation.
Problem solving	Identification of problems and possible solutions.
Stress tolerance	Adaptation and coping in the midst of stress.

Impulse control	Delaying or resisting an impulse.
Optimism	Looking at the bright side, maintaining a positive attitude.
Happiness	Satisfaction with life, the ability to enjoy self and others.

Source: Bar On 1997.

About the Author

ESTELLE CODIER is an associate professor at the University of Hawai'i's School of Nursing. She is the author of more than two dozen peer-reviewed articles and has made both national and international presentations and workshops on MUVE learning. Professor Codier has supervised more than 400 learning activities in Second Life® and continues to use MUVE learning in both undergraduate and graduate courses, some of which take place entirely in Second Life®.